THERAPEUTIC EXERCISES

using the

SWISS BALL

Caroline Corning Creager, P.T.

EXECUTIVE PHYSICAL THERAPY

BOULDER, COLORADO

Library of Congress Card Catalog Number: 94-94327
Creager, Caroline Corning
        Therapeutic Exercises Using the Swiss Ball.
        Creager, Caroline Corning – 1st edition, 3rd printing.

                                Executive Physical Therapy, Inc.
                                P.O. Box 1319
                                Berthoud, CO 80513

                                1-800-530-6878.

The author has made every effort to assure that the information in this book is
accurate and current at the time of printing. The publisher and author take no
responsibilities for the use of the material in this book and cannot be held
responsible for any typographical or other errors found.

ISBN: 0-9651153-0-1
Library of Congress Card Catalog Number: 94-94327

Book design by Caroline Corning Creager
Composition by Alan Bernhard
Cover design by Paulette Livers Lambert
Illustrations by Mike Berry
Hand illustrations by Cathy Davenport
Edited by Caryl Riedel

                        Distributed by:
                          OPTP
            P.O. Box 47009, Minneapolis, MN 55447, USA
                (612) 553-0452   (800) 367-7393

About the Author

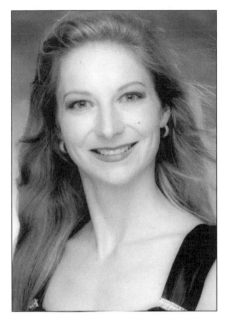

© Marc Nader, 1994

C aroline Corning Creager was born in Richmond,
Virginia, and raised in Wasilla, Alaska. She received a
Bachelor of Science in Physical Therapy from the
University of Montana in 1989. She is the owner of
Executive Physical Therapy, Inc. in Boulder, Colorado, and
instructs at Pima Medical Institute in Denver, Colorado.
She teaches seminars entitled "Therapeutic Exercises Using
the Swiss Ball" throughout the United States.

Dedication

To my husband Robert, who has given new meaning to my
   life.

To my parents, Mary and Raymond Corning, and to my
   sister and brother, Muriel and Vincent Corning, who
   have given me unwavering love and support
   throughout my life.

To Janet Sorensen, L.P.T. and Alice Holinger, L.P.T., who
   gave me the inspiration to become a physical
   therapist.

To the State of Alaska, where I grew up, and the State of
   Colorado, where I now reside.

Acknowledgments

To Patricia Toillion, O.T.R., for her friendship and valuable suggestions in helping me write and teach the exercises presented in this book.

To Diane Blanchard, P.T., and Ann Dawdy, P.T., for offering valuable suggestions and editing the manuscript.

To Doug Dewey, P.T., O.C.S., for his dedication to the field of physical therapy.

To Mark Barnes, M.P.T., for giving me the opportunity to share my treatment philosophies.

To Mike Berry, for devoting all his free hours to illustrating this book.

To Alan Bernhard, for helping me make the best book possible.

Footprints

ONE NIGHT I HAD A DREAM —
I dreamed I was walking along the beach with the Lord,
and across the sky flashed scenes from my life.
For each scene I noticed two sets of footprints in the sand:
one belonged to me and the other to the Lord.

When the last scene of my life flashed before me, I looked back
at the footprints in the sand. I noticed that many times along
the path of my life, there was only one set of footprints. I also
noticed that it happened at the very lowest and saddest times
of my life.

This really bothered me, and I questioned the Lord about it.

"Lord, you said that once I decided to follow you, you would
walk with me all the way. But I have noticed that during the
most troublesome times in my life, there is only one set of
footprints. I don't understand why in times when I needed
you most, you should leave me."

The Lord replied, "My precious child, I love you and would
never ever leave you during your times of trial and suffering.
When you saw only one set of footprints, it was then that I
carried you."

– Author Unknown

Foreword

Exercise is an integral part of the progressive treatment approach for musculoskeletal dysfunction. We as health care providers must, in some capacity, facilitate the return of quality, pain-free movement in our patients. This process is best accomplished through education that is experiential for the patient. The avenues for this have been varied. The Swiss Ball has proved to be an excellent tool for motor reeducation in neurological and orthopedic rehabilitation.

Caroline's presentation on this topic has exemplified her deep understanding of facilitated exercise. This collection of exercises is well-rounded and encompasses dynamic spinal stability with extremity work. The three-dimensional aspect of the figures gives a clear depiction of position, technique, and kinetics of the desired exercise. The page layout allows for appropriate, concise information for the patient and therapist. This clarity is critical for the success of therapeutic instruction and patient independence with the exercise.

Mark F. Barnes, M.P.T.

Preface

The need for an illustrated text with Swiss Ball Exercises became apparent after hand writing instructions for my patients' Swiss Ball Exercise Programs. Hand writing exercises is inefficient and time-consuming for me. This book provides more than 250 illustrated exercises for the therapist to photocopy for patient use and create a comprehensive Swiss Ball exercise program.

Each drawing was specifically designed to add a three-dimensional effect. Shading was used to depict movement of the ball and body.

Exercises were categorized by body position on the ball, and listed by common and technical names. The PURPOSE of the exercises and the INSTRUCTIONS were written in laymen's terms. Each page provides a SPECIAL PROTOCOLS/NOTES section to allow the therapist to modify the exercise and individualize each patient program.

The focus of this book is to improve individualized clinical, work, and home exercise programs by providing illustrated and easy-to-read instructions. I hope to expand each therapist's repertoire of exercises and encourage therapists to create new exercises that facilitate the needs of their patients.

From personal experience in instructing independent home exercise programs, I have found that patient compliance is greater when the patient uses a Swiss Ball and has instructions. In addition, the following cues may help improve patient compliance and retention: verbally instruct patient, demonstrate the exercise, ask patient to visualize and then perform exercise, and lastly, have patient recite the instructions and repeat the exercise.

Caroline Corning Creager, P.T.

Table of Contents

History of the Swiss Ball

Originally, large, inflatable vinyl balls were used in the 1960s by Swiss physiotherapists to help children with cerebral palsy facilitate balance and equilibrium reactions, hence, the name Swiss Ball. Frau Susanne Klein-Vogelbach, former Head of the Physiotherapy School of the Kantonsspital in Basel, Switzerland, was one of the first therapists to begin using the Swiss Ball as a therapeutic tool.[1, 2] She incorporated the use of the ball into treatment regimens for neurologic and orthopedic patients.

In Europe, the use of the ball and Functional Kinetics are taught in almost every physiotherapy school as basic "reactive exercises," according to Isabelle Gloor-Moriconi, a Swiss physiotherapist. Frau Klein-Vogelbach lectured on the benefits of Functional Kinetics and its application to the ball for many years. At the age of 83, Frau Klein-Vogelbach continues to teach Swiss Ball and Functional Kinetics techniques in Basel, Switzerland.

In 1972, Maria Kucera, a Czechoslovakian physical therapist, attended one of Frau Klein-Vogelbach's Functional Kinetics courses and was inspired to adopt the use of the Swiss Ball. When Maria Kucera returned to the Zurich Physical Therapy School where she taught, she began using the Swiss Ball with her students and patients. As a result, Ms. Kucera published a book entitled *Gymnastic mit dem Hupfball*.[3] This book has been a resource for European physical therapists since 1973.

Caroline Creager has written and published three books, *Therapeutic Exercises Using the Swiss Ball*, *Caroline Creager's Airobic Ball™ Strengthening Workout*, and *Caroline Creager's Airobic Ball™ Stretching Workout*. Caroline lectures and teaches seminars throughout the United States promoting Swiss Ball techniques.

The following therapists throughout the United States have been influential in the instruction of the Swiss Ball: Barbara Headley, Dennis Morgan, Beate Carriere, Barbara Hypes, Nancy Good, Joanne Posner-Mayer, and Kathie Hanson.

Ninoska Gomez, Ph.D., reported that "rolling, turning, and balancing on them (the balls) provides a great deal of tactile and vestibular stimulation which activates and helps integrate the reflexes, righting reactions, and equilibrium reactions."[4]

Darcy Umphred, Ph.D., R.P.T., stated that "having a client sitting on a ball doing almost any exercise will stimulate vestibular and proprioceptive responses."[5]

Ball activities add diversification to treatment regimens and are enjoyed by all ages and patient populations. The following patient populations have been successfully treated with the Swiss Ball: pediatric, postpartum, geriatric, orthopedic, neurologic, cardiac, chronic pain, and sports medicine. Swiss Balls can be found in almost every physical therapy department in the United States and continue to gain in popularity.

Introduction

DETERMINING APPROPRIATE BALL SIZE

To better understand the exercises presented in this book, each therapist should be able to demonstrate the exercises before administering to the patient. Please keep in mind that each patient's body proportions are different and, therefore, each exercise may need to be adapted to each individual patient.[6] The recommended ball sizes and inflation techniques serve only as guidelines. Dr. Susanne Klein-Vogelbach wrote, "To overcome deficits in the patient's movement behavior, it is not the patient who must adapt to the exercise, but the exercise that must be adapted to the patient."[7]

Ball size is determined by patient height and weight, intended exercise position (prone, supine, sitting, etc.) and the goals of treatment. A smaller ball (30 cm. or 45 cm.) has less surface area, requiring more energy to maintain balance. The small ball may be indicated for an athletic patient or for a patient with a total knee replacement to promote increased range of motion.

A large ball has greater surface area and, therefore, may be indicated for the overweight or involved patient, for patients requiring upper extremity weight bearing, or to enable the patient and the therapist to sit on the ball together.

A fully inflated or firm ball has less contact area on the floor, moves more quickly, and, therefore, challenges balance reactions more than an underinflated ball. An underinflated or soft ball has greater contact area, moves more slowly, and, therefore, requires less energy to maintain balance.

References have been made to a "mini" ball and "small" ball throughout this book. A mini ball measures 40 to 55 milli-

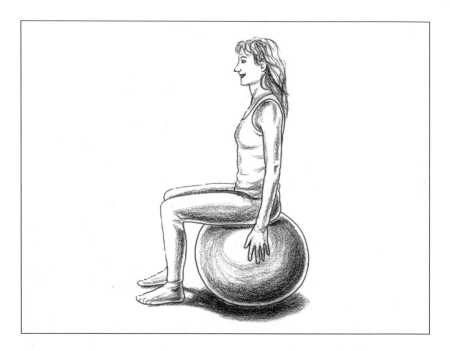

meters (smaller than a racquet ball), and a small ball measures 30 centimeters in diameter.

Ideally, if a patient is sitting on the ball with feet flat, the hips and knees should form a 90 degree angle.

The following serves as a guideline in determining the appropriate ball size for exercises in sitting.

30 cm. ball	children 1 – 2 years old
45 cm. ball	< 5'0" tall
55 cm. ball	5'0" to 5'7" tall
65 cm. ball	5'8" to 6'3" tall
75 cm. ball	> 6'3" tall

In the supine position, if the ball is placed under the knees, the ball height should equal the distance between the greater trochanter and the joint line of the knee.

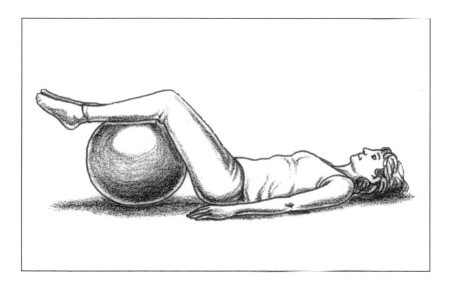

In the quadriped position, the ball height should equal the distance between the shoulder and wrist.

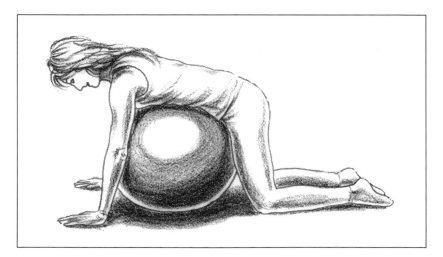

Generally, the ball size required for the bridge position is the same as for sitting.

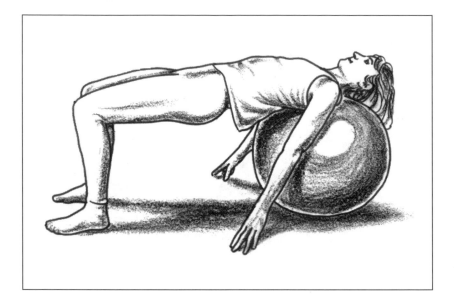

Ball Care Instructions

Proper Inflation Techniques

Allow the ball to reach room temperature before inflating. The balls inflate to a variety of maximum diameters (i.e., 45 cm., 55 cm., etc.) and the maximum diameter is usually printed on the ball. The differing ball diameters allow inflation of balls to approximately the same rigidity and allow for differing measurements in overall diameter. It is imperative that the recommended maximum diameter for a given size not be exceeded.

To measure the diameter of the ball, take a yard stick and place on top of the ball. Place a tape measure on the floor and measure up to the yard stick. A second method requires measuring from the floor up the wall 55 cm. (or the appropriate maximum diameter for each ball) and putting a pencil mark on the wall. Inflate the ball up to the pencil mark.

Many methods are available for inflating the Swiss Ball:

1. air compressor
2. hand pump
3. raft pump
4. air mattress pump
5. tire pump with a trigger nozzle adapter

The air compressor forces compressed air into the ball, quickly inflating the ball. (Be careful not to overinflate the ball.) The air compressor may be one of the easiest ways to inflate a ball. Many hospital maintenance departments use air compressors and, therefore, can assist with inflating the balls.

Hand, raft, and mattress pumps are inexpensive and can be purchased for home or clinic use. Tire pumps at local gas stations can be used in conjunction with a trigger nozzle adapter to inflate the balls. Bicycle pumps are inefficient and not powerful enough to properly inflate the balls.

Every three to four months the balls may require additional air. If the balls are used extensively, air may need to be added more frequently.

PROPER CLEANING TECHNIQUES

Clean the balls with soap and water at home. In the clinic, use infection control agents between patients in order to prevent cross contamination.

PROTOCOLS FOR USING THE SWISS BALL

INDICATIONS

1. decreased range of motion
2. decreased strength
3. decreased balance reactions
4. decreased coordination
5. decreased endurance
6. decreased proprioception
7. decreased cardiovascular fitness
8. decreased flexibility in myofascial and scar tissue

PRECAUTIONS

1. muscular fatigue
2. cardiovascular distress
   a. shortness of breath
   b. light-headedness
   c. pallor
   d. nausea
   e. angina
3. adhering to weight restrictions (i.e., non-weight bearing, partial weight bearing, etc.)
4. aggravating degenerative joint disease with mobility exercises
5. following specific injury precautions (i.e., do not exceed 90 degrees of hip flexion with new total hip replacement patients)
6. superseding patient tolerance level
7. signs of sensory overload
   a. pupil dilation
   b. sweaty palms
   c. changes in respiration rate
   d. flushing or pallor
   e. complaints of dizziness

CONTRAINDICATIONS

1. increase in pain
2. dizziness/nausea
3. ringing in ears
4. ball activities frighten patient

Helpful Hints

1. The further away the ball is from the body the more difficult the exercise.
   ex. Exercise # 124 is more difficult than exercise # 122.

2. The further away the extremities are from the ball, the more difficult the exercise.
   ex. Exercise # 200 is more difficult than exercise # 199.

3. Normal gait speed is between .91 and 1.52 meters/second or between 112 and 120 steps per minute.[9] The goal for an exercise simulating gait should be normal gait speed.
   ex. a. Do 112 to 120 bounces per minute for exercise # 49.
   *   b. Take 112 to 120 steps per minute for exercise # 72.*

4. Adding a bounce to the exercise makes the exercise more challenging.

5. Visual cues may be added to better facilitate therapist and patient techniques.
   a. Place a mirror in front of patient and/or therapist.
   b. Tape "X"s on the floor so patient has visual stimuli as to where to put the feet.

6. Closing the eyes increases the difficulty of the exercise.

7. Provide patient with manual resistance when on the ball.

8. Add resistance with cuff or free weights.

9. The color of the ball may be important: bright colors activate the central nervous system and increase tone. Dark colors help to decrease tone.[8]

10. Children or adults who are fearful of the prone position on the ball may benefit from a clear ball. The clear ball allows the child/adult to see the floor.

11. The physio*roll* shape restricts side to side movement and provides a larger surface area. The physioroll allows two people to sit on the ball together and permits upper extremity weight bearing in sitting.

12. Vinyl balls hold up to 300 kilograms or 660 pounds of force; balls made out of P.V.C. foam hold up to 200 kilograms or 440 pounds of force.

13. A variety of mediums may be added to the inside of the balls (beans, rice, water, mini balls, and sand) to promote different sensorimotor responses.

14. Remind patients to do exercises at home away from furniture and sharp objects.

Stretching

Proper stretching techniques are essential to effectively increase the length of connective tissue. Try to design stretching programs to be performed 15–20 minutes before exercising and once again thereafter.[10] Individualize the stretching program to injury-specific diagnoses and to activities in which the patient engages (athletics, work, etc.).

To properly stretch a muscle, maintain a slow static stretch. Bouncing or sudden stretching of a muscle excites the muscle spindle, sending signals to the spinal cord which then transmits signals back down to the extrafusal muscle fibers causing a reflex contraction of the muscle being stretched. This contraction is referred to as the myotatic reflex or stretch reflex. The stretch reflex protects our muscles from being overstretched or injured.

The following guidelines were adapted from "The Warm-up Procedure: To Stretch or Not to Stretch. A Brief Review," by Craig Smith.[11]

1. Avoid bouncing.

2. Apply a slow static stretch into level of tolerance, not pain.

3. Hold stretch for 15–20 seconds.

4. Release stretch slowly.

5. Repeat stretch to each muscle group three to five times.

6. Alternate stretching agonistic and antagonistic muscle groups.

A Stretching Information Sheet written for the patient has been included; please see page 16.

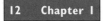

Reimbursement

M any private insurance companies will reimburse the patient for the cost of the Swiss Ball if the patient acquires a prescription from his/her doctor indicating medical necessity. Health Maintenance Organizations and Preferred Provider Organizations are less likely to reimburse the expense of a Swiss Ball. One basic guideline to follow is, if the insurance company reimburses for medical equipment or medical supplies, the company is more likely to cover the expense of a Swiss Ball.

Workman's Compensation policies vary greatly from state to state, however, in most cases, Workman's Compensation will reimburse the patient for the Swiss Ball expense. Medicare will not cover the cost of a Swiss Ball.

Proper billing documentation is an essential component of reimbursement for medical supplies. The correct code number for billing purposes of the Swiss Ball is: 99070. Swiss Balls vary in size, shape, medium, and price. Therefore, include the size of the Swiss Ball (45 cm., 55 cm., 65 cm., etc.), the type of ball (roll, ball, PVC foam, etc.), and the price ($49.95, $14.95, $24.95, etc.) in the medical supply description.

The following is an example of billing documentation:

Date of Service	Procedure Code #	Describe supplies furnished for each date given	Charges
5/3/94	99070	Physioroll 55 cm.	$49.95
5/3/94	99070	Swiss Ball 45 cm.	$14.95
5/3/94	99070	Swiss Ball 65 cm. (PVC foam)	$24.95

Over the last five years health care costs have risen and Swiss Ball prices have fallen. Accordingly, patients who are not reimbursed by their insurance companies are now able to purchase and incorporate the Swiss Ball into their individualized home exercise program.

Notes

1. Klein-Vogelbach, Susanne. *Therapeutic Exercises in Functional Kinetics.* Springer-Verlag, Germany, 1991.
2. Kucera, Maria. *Gymnastik mit dem Hupfball.* Gustav Fisher Verlag, Stuttgart, 1978.
3. Hypes, Barbara. *Facilitating Development and Sensorimotor Function: Treatment with the Ball.* PDP Press, Minnesota, 1991.
4. Gomez, Niska. "Somarhythms: Developing Somatic Awareness with Large, Inflatable Balls." *Somatics.* Spring/Summer, 1992. pp. 12–18.
5. Umphred, Darcy Ann. *Neurological Rehabilitation.* C.V. Mosby Company, Missouri, 1985.
6. Carriere, Beate. "In Consideration of Proportions." *PT Magazine.* April, 1993. pp. 56–61.
7. Klein-Vogelbach, Susanne. *Therapeutic Exercises in Functional Kinetics.* Springer-Verlag, Germany, 1991.
8. Umphred, Darcy Ann. *Neurological Rehabilitation.* C.V. Mosby Company, Missouri, 1985.
9. Davies, Patricia. *Right in the Middle: Selective Trunk Activity in the Treatment of Adult Hemiplegia.* Springer-Verlag, Germany, 1990.
10. Smith, Craig. "The Warm-up Procedure: To Stretch or Not to Stretch. A Brief Review." *J. Ortho. Sports Phys. Ther.* 19(1):12–17, 1994.
11. Smith, Craig. "The Warm-up Procedure: To Stretch or Not to Stretch. A Brief Review." *J. Ortho. Sports Phys. Ther.* 19(1):12–17, 1994.

CHAPTER TWO
Stretching

Stretching Techniques

PURPOSE: To safely and effectively increase muscle length.

INSTRUCTIONS: 1. Avoid bouncing.

2. Slowly stretch into level of tolerance, not pain.

3. Do not hold your breath.

4. Repeat stretch <u>three</u> to <u>five</u> times.

5. Repeat on both sides of body.

SPECIAL PROTOCOLS/NOTES: _____

_____

_____

PATIENT NAME: _____DATE:_____

THERAPIST NAME:_____

Cervical Side Bend Stretch

PURPOSE: To stretch neck muscles.

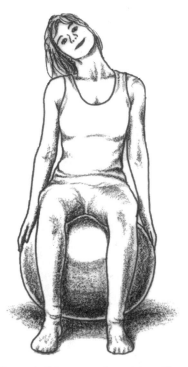

INSTRUCTION: Sit on ball in neutral position. Keep head/ears in line with shoulders. Bend head sideways toward shoulder. Repeat on opposite side.

Hold: _____ second(s).   Repeat: _____ time(s).

Frequency: _____ x/day.

SPECIAL PROTOCOLS/NOTES: _____

_____

_____

PATIENT NAME: _____DATE:_____

THERAPIST NAME:_____

Cervical Rotation Stretch

PURPOSE: To increase range of motion in neck.

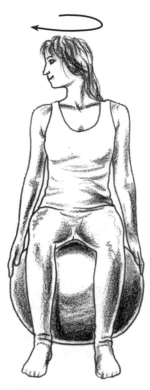

INSTRUCTION: Sit on ball in neutral position. Place hands on side of ball. Rotate head slowly to the right and look over shoulder. Repeat to the left.

Hold: _____ second(s).   Repeat: _____ time(s).

Frequency: _____ x/day.

SPECIAL PROTOCOLS/NOTES: _____

_____

_____

PATIENT NAME: _____DATE:_____

THERAPIST NAME:_____

Cervical Rotation Stretch

PURPOSE: To stretch neck muscles.

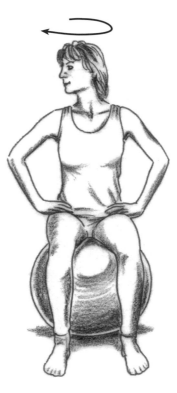

INSTRUCTION: Sit on ball in neutral position. Place hands on hips. Rotate head slowly to the right, look over shoulder. Repeat to the left.

Hold: _____ second(s).   Repeat: _____ time(s).

Frequency: _____ x/day.

SPECIAL PROTOCOLS/NOTES: Keep shoulders relaxed. _____

_____

_____

PATIENT NAME: _____DATE:_____

THERAPIST NAME:_____

Levator Scapulae Stretch

PURPOSE: To stretch neck muscles.

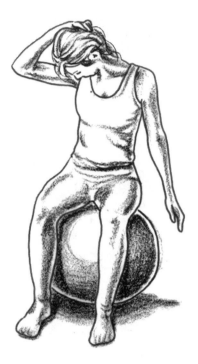

INSTRUCTION: Sit on ball. Place right hand behind head. Extend left arm slightly behind back and reach for floor. Bend neck forward and look down at right knee. Repeat with left hand and right arm.

Hold: _____ second(s).   Repeat: _____ time(s).

Frequency: _____ x/day.

SPECIAL PROTOCOLS/NOTES: _____

_____

_____

PATIENT NAME: _____DATE:_____

THERAPIST NAME:_____

Anterior Foot Stretch

PURPOSE: To stretch front of foot muscles.

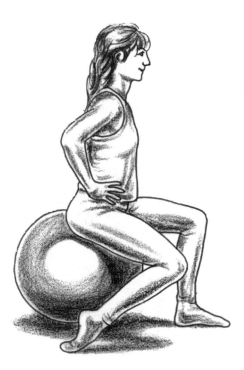

INSTRUCTION: Sit on ball in neutral position. Point toe and move foot back beside ball so top of foot faces downward. Repeat with opposite side.

Hold: _____ second(s).   Repeat: _____ time(s).

Frequency: _____ x/day.

SPECIAL PROTOCOLS/NOTES: _____

_____

_____

PATIENT NAME: _____ DATE: _____

THERAPIST NAME: _____

Soleus Stretch

PURPOSE: To stretch shin muscles.

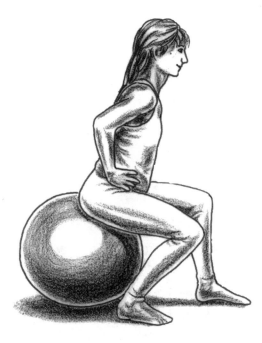

INSTRUCTION: Sit on ball in neutral position. Move one foot back beside ball. Lean forward at waist. Repeat with opposite side.

Hold: _____ second(s).   Repeat: _____ time(s).

Frequency: _____ x/day.

SPECIAL PROTOCOLS/NOTES: _Keep heel down during exercise._____

_____

_____

PATIENT NAME: _____DATE:_____

THERAPIST NAME:_____

Hamstring and Calf Stretch

PURPOSE: To stretch hamstring muscles.

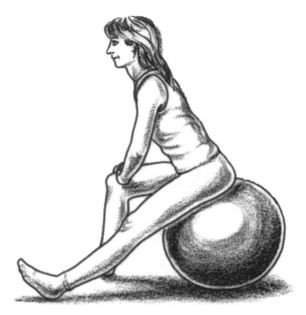

INSTRUCTION: Sit on ball in neutral position. Lean forward. Straighten leg. Place hands on bent knee. Straighten opposite leg. Pull toes up toward ceiling. Repeat with opposite side.

Hold: _____ second(s).   Repeat: _____ time(s).

Frequency: _____ x/day.

SPECIAL PROTOCOLS/NOTES: _Keep head up. Try to keep back in_
_neutral position._____

_____

PATIENT NAME: _____ DATE:_____

THERAPIST NAME:_____

Hip Flexor Stretch - I

PURPOSE: To stretch hip muscles.

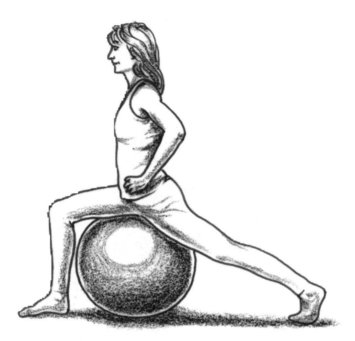

INSTRUCTION: Sit on ball in neutral position. Slide one leg behind ball. Straighten back leg. Keep front leg bent. Repeat with opposite side.

Hold: _____ second(s).   Repeat: _____ time(s).

Frequency: _____ x/day.

SPECIAL PROTOCOLS/NOTES: _Do not arch back._ _____

_____

_____

PATIENT NAME: _____DATE:_____

THERAPIST NAME:_____

Hip Flexor Stretch - II

PURPOSE: To increase range of motion in hips.

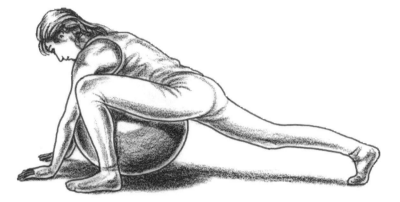

INSTRUCTION: Kneel. Lunge forward with one bent knee. Place ball under abdomen, reach one leg back and straighten. Repeat with opposite side.

Hold: _____ second(s).   Repeat: _____ time(s).

Frequency: _____ x/day.

SPECIAL PROTOCOLS/NOTES: _____

_____

_____

PATIENT NAME: _____ DATE:_____

THERAPIST NAME:_____

Quadricep Stretch

PURPOSE: To stretch quadricep muscles.

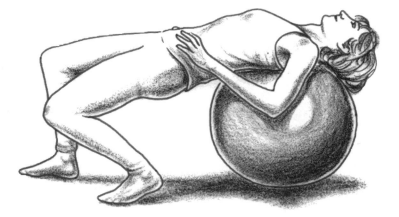

INSTRUCTION: Sit on ball. Walk feet out so head and shoulders rest on ball. Slide one heel back toward head. Repeat with opposite side.

Hold: _____ second(s).   Repeat: _____ time(s).

Frequency: _____ x/day.

SPECIAL PROTOCOLS/NOTES: __Do not let buttocks sag._____

_____

_____

PATIENT NAME: _____DATE:_____

THERAPIST NAME:_____

Unilateral Hip Adductor Stretch

PURPOSE: To increase range of motion in inside of thighs.

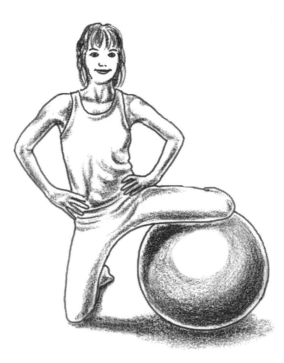

INSTRUCTION: Kneel. Place one bent knee on top of ball. Repeat with opposite knee.

Hold: _____ second(s).   Repeat: _____ time(s).

Frequency: _____ x/day.

SPECIAL PROTOCOLS/NOTES: _____

_____

_____

PATIENT NAME: _____ DATE: _____

THERAPIST NAME: _____

Bilateral Hip Adductor Stretch

PURPOSE: To increase range of motion in inside of thighs.

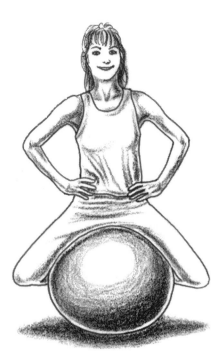

INSTRUCTION: Sit on ball. Slide one knee around to side of ball. Slide second knee around side of ball. Toes touch floor behind ball.

Hold: _____ second(s).   Repeat: _____ time(s).

Frequency: _____ x/day.

SPECIAL PROTOCOLS/NOTES: _____

_____

_____

PATIENT NAME: _____DATE:_____

THERAPIST NAME:_____

Sidelying Stretch—
Superior Leg Extended

PURPOSE: To stretch muscles in torso.

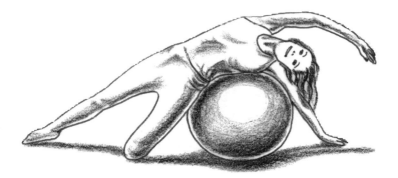

INSTRUCTION: Kneel. Place ball alongside of body. Stretch over ball with arm overhead. Keep bottom leg bent. Straighten top leg. Repeat with opposite side.

Hold: _____ second(s).   Repeat: _____ time(s).

Frequency: _____ x/day.

SPECIAL PROTOCOLS/NOTES: _____

_____

_____

PATIENT NAME: _____DATE:_____

THERAPIST NAME:_____

Sidelying Stretch—
Superior Knee Flexed

PURPOSE: To stretch muscles in torso.

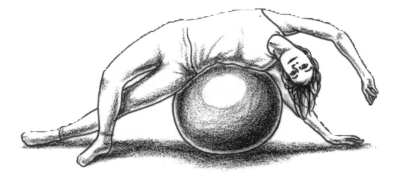

INSTRUCTION: Kneel. Place ball alongside of body. Stretch over ball with arm overhead. Straighten bottom leg and cross top leg over bottom leg. Repeat with opposite side.

Hold: _____ second(s).   Repeat: _____ time(s).

Frequency: _____ x/day.

SPECIAL PROTOCOLS/NOTES: _____

_____

_____

PATIENT NAME: _____DATE:_____

THERAPIST NAME:_____

Brachioplexus Stretch

PURPOSE: To stretch shoulder and chest muscles.

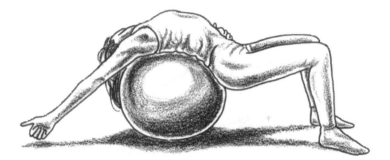

INSTRUCTION: Sit on ball. Walk feet out so head and shoulders are resting on ball. Stretch arm overhead and rotate hand so palm is facing ceiling. Rotate head in opposite direction. Repeat with opposite arm.

Hold: _____ second(s).   Repeat: _____ time(s).

Frequency: _____ x/day.

SPECIAL PROTOCOLS/NOTES: _____

_____

_____

PATIENT NAME: _____DATE:_____

THERAPIST NAME:_____

Trunk Extension Stretch

PURPOSE: To stretch arm, leg, back, and neck muscles.

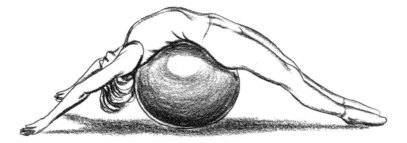

INSTRUCTION: Lie on ball in bridge position. Raise arms overhead and straighten legs out.

Hold: _____ second(s).   Repeat: _____ time(s).

Frequency: _____ x/day.

SPECIAL PROTOCOLS/NOTES: _____

_____

_____

PATIENT NAME: _____ DATE: _____

THERAPIST NAME: _____

Prone Body Flexion Stretch

PURPOSE: To increase flexibility in back and neck.

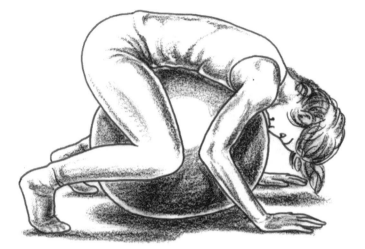

INSTRUCTION: Lie with abdomen on ball. Bend knees and place on each side of ball. Bend elbows and relax head down.

Hold: _____ second(s).   Repeat: _____ time(s).

Frequency: _____ x/day.

SPECIAL PROTOCOLS/NOTES: _____

_____ _____

_____

PATIENT NAME: _____DATE:_____

THERAPIST NAME:_____

Bilateral Shoulder Flexion Stretch

PURPOSE: To increase range of motion in shoulders.

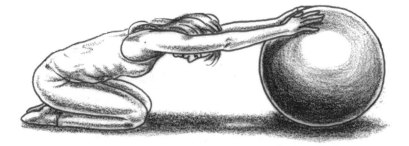

INSTRUCTION: Kneel. Sit back on heels. Roll ball away from body. Keep hands on ball. Keep arms straight.

Hold: _____ second(s).   Repeat: _____ time(s).

Frequency: _____ x/day.

SPECIAL PROTOCOLS/NOTES: _____

_____

_____

PATIENT NAME: _____DATE:_____

THERAPIST NAME:_____

Bilateral Shoulder Roll Stretch

PURPOSE: To increase range of motion in shoulders.

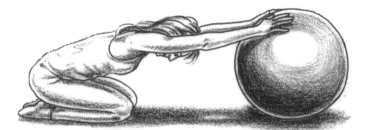

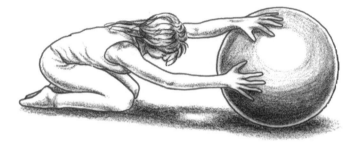

INSTRUCTION: Kneel. Sit back on heels. Roll ball away from body. Keep hands on ball. Keep arms straight. Roll ball from side to side.

Hold: _____ second(s).   Repeat: _____ time(s).

Frequency: _____ x/day.

SPECIAL PROTOCOLS/NOTES: _____

_____

_____

PATIENT NAME: _____ DATE:_____

THERAPIST NAME:_____

Unilateral Shoulder Roll Stretch

PURPOSE: To increase range of motion and strengthen shoulder muscles.

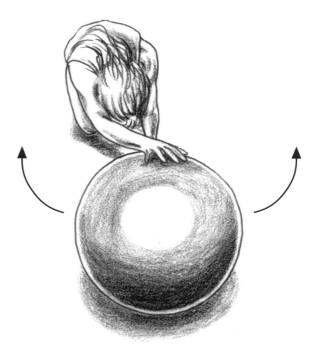

INSTRUCTION: Kneel. Sit back on heels. Roll ball away from body. Keep hand on ball. Keep arm straight. Roll ball from side to side. Repeat with opposite side.

Hold: _____ second(s).   Repeat: _____ time(s).

Frequency: _____ x/day.

SPECIAL PROTOCOLS/NOTES: _____

_____

_____

PATIENT NAME: _____ DATE: _____

THERAPIST NAME: _____

Shoulder Mobilization Stretch

PURPOSE: To increase range of motion in shoulders.

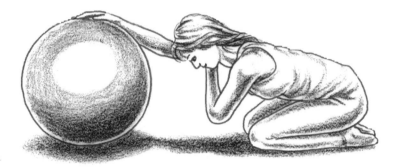

INSTRUCTION: Kneel. Place right hand on ball. Place left hand on right shoulder. Lean forward. Repeat with opposite side.

Hold: _____ second(s).   Repeat: _____ time(s).

Frequency: _____ x/day.

SPECIAL PROTOCOLS/NOTES: Keep back straight. _____

_____

_____

PATIENT NAME: _____ DATE:_____

THERAPIST NAME:_____

Standing Shoulder Flexion Stretch

PURPOSE: To stretch shoulder muscles.

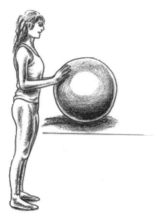
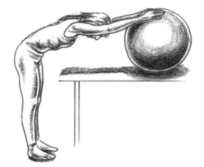

INSTRUCTION: Stand. Place ball on table and hands on top of ball. Straighten arms, push ball forward, and lean body forward.

Hold: _____ second(s).   Repeat: _____ time(s).

Frequency: _____ x/day.

SPECIAL PROTOCOLS/NOTES: Do not arch back. _____

_____

_____

PATIENT NAME: _____ DATE: _____

THERAPIST NAME: _____

Metatarsal and Phalangeal Stretch

PURPOSE: To stretch toes and arch of foot.

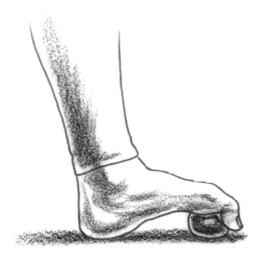

INSTRUCTION: Sit in chair. Place mini ball on floor. Curl toes around mini ball. Repeat with opposite side.

Hold: _____ second(s).   Repeat: _____ time(s).

Frequency: _____ x/day.

SPECIAL PROTOCOLS/NOTES: _____

_____

_____

PATIENT NAME: _____DATE:_____

THERAPIST NAME:_____

CHAPTER THREE
Sitting

Neutral Position in Sitting

PURPOSE: To strengthen muscles in an optimal position to avoid injury.

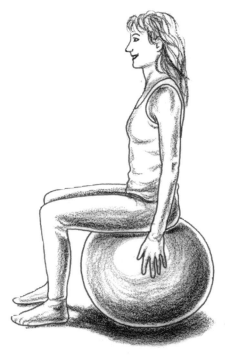

INSTRUCTION: Sit on ball with toes pointing forward. Align knees over feet. Maintain natural curve in back.

Hold: _____ second(s).   Repeat: _____ time(s).

Frequency: _____ x/day.

SPECIAL PROTOCOLS/NOTES: _Do not arch back or slouch._____

_____

_____

PATIENT NAME: _____DATE:_____

THERAPIST NAME:_____

Cervical Flexion Press

PURPOSE: To strengthen neck muscles.

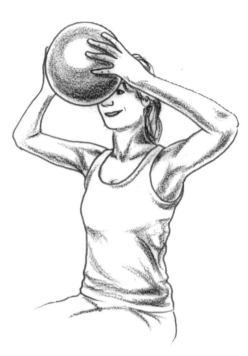

INSTRUCTION: Sit on ball in neutral position. Place small ball on forehead. Lightly press forehead into ball.

Hold: _____ second(s).   Repeat: _____ time(s).

Frequency: _____ x/day.

SPECIAL PROTOCOLS/NOTES: _____

_____   _____

_____

PATIENT NAME: _____DATE:_____

THERAPIST NAME:_____

Cervical Extension Press

PURPOSE: To strengthen neck muscles.

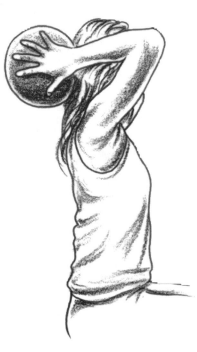

INSTRUCTION: Sit on ball in neutral position. Place ball behind head. Lightly press head into ball.

Hold: _____ second(s).   Repeat: _____ time(s).

Frequency: _____ x/day.

SPECIAL PROTOCOLS/NOTES: _____

_____

_____

PATIENT NAME: _____DATE:_____

THERAPIST NAME:_____

Cervical Lateral Flexion Press

PURPOSE: To strengthen neck muscles.

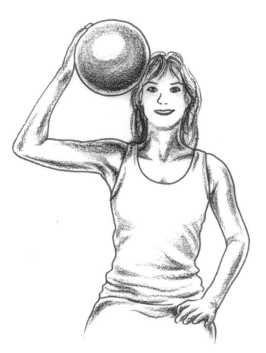

INSTRUCTION: Sit on ball in neutral position. Place small ball against side of head. Lightly press head into ball. Repeat on opposite side.

Hold: _____ second(s).   Repeat: _____ time(s).

Frequency: _____ x/day.

SPECIAL PROTOCOLS/NOTES: _____

_____

_____

PATIENT NAME: _____ DATE: _____

THERAPIST NAME: _____

Cervical Rotation Press

PURPOSE: To strengthen neck muscles.

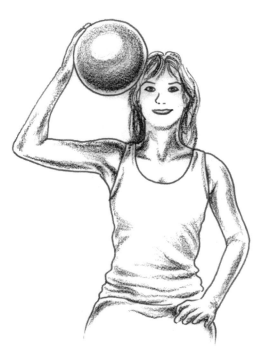

INSTRUCTION: Sit on ball in neutral position. Place small ball on right side of head. Lightly press head into ball. Turn head to right. Repeat on opposite side.

Hold: _____ second(s).   Repeat: _____ time(s).

Frequency: _____ x/day.

SPECIAL PROTOCOLS/NOTES: _____

_____

_____

PATIENT NAME: _____ DATE: _____

THERAPIST NAME: _____

Bounce on Ball

PURPOSE: To increase nutrition to discs in neck and back. To improve coordination.

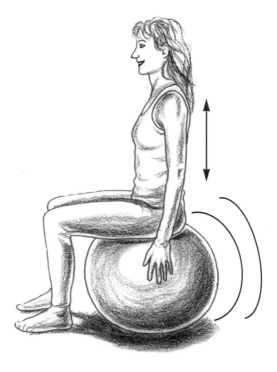

INSTRUCTION: Sit on ball in neutral position. Bounce on ball.

Hold: _____ second(s).   Repeat: _____ time(s).

Frequency: _____ x/day.

SPECIAL PROTOCOLS/NOTES: ___Do not hold breath. Exhale when___
___buttocks make contact with ball._____

_____

PATIENT NAME: _____DATE:_____

THERAPIST NAME:_____

Anterior Pelvic Tilt

PURPOSE: To increase flexibility in back and hips.

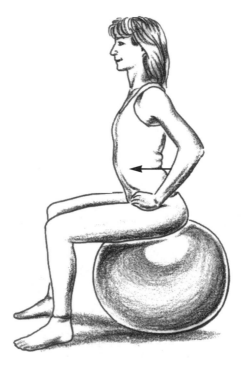

INSTRUCTION: Sit on ball in neutral position. Roll ball backward as hips roll forward. Slightly arch back. Return to neutral position.

Hold: _____ second(s).   Repeat: _____ time(s).

Frequency: _____ x/day.

SPECIAL PROTOCOLS/NOTES: _____

_____

_____

PATIENT NAME: _____ DATE: _____

THERAPIST NAME: _____

Posterior Pelvic Tilt

PURPOSE: To increase flexibility in back and hips.

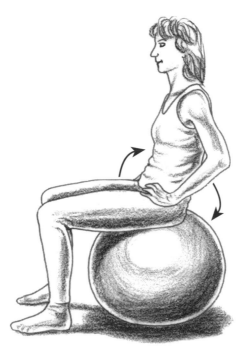

INSTRUCTION: Sit on ball in neutral position. Roll ball forward as hips roll backward. Return to neutral position.

Hold: _____ second(s).   Repeat: _____ time(s).

Frequency: _____ x/day.

SPECIAL PROTOCOLS/NOTES: _____

_____

_____

PATIENT NAME: _____ DATE:_____

THERAPIST NAME:_____

Lateral Weight Shift

PURPOSE: To lengthen and strengthen trunk muscles. To encourage shifting body weight equally from side to side.

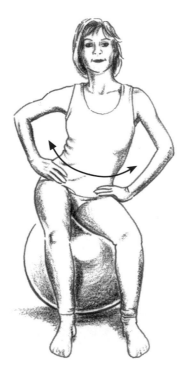

INSTRUCTION: Sit on ball in neutral position. Roll ball from side to side by shifting weight from right hip to left hip.

Hold: _____ second(s).   Repeat: _____ time(s).

Frequency: _____ x/day.

SPECIAL PROTOCOLS/NOTES: _____

_____

_____

PATIENT NAME: _____DATE:_____

THERAPIST NAME:_____

Lateral Weight Shift with Thoracic Spine Stabilized

PURPOSE: To lengthen and strengthen trunk muscles. To encourage shifting body weight equally from side to side.

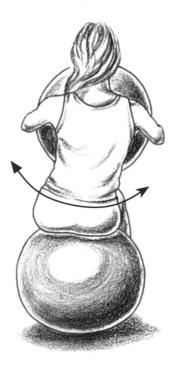

INSTRUCTION: Sit on ball in neutral position. Place second ball in arms. Hug ball. Roll first ball from side to side by shifting weight from right hip to left hip.

Hold: _____ second(s).   Repeat: _____ time(s).

Frequency: _____ x/day.

SPECIAL PROTOCOLS/NOTES: _____

_____

_____

PATIENT NAME: _____DATE:_____

THERAPIST NAME:_____

Pelvic Circles

PURPOSE: To increase back and hip flexibility.

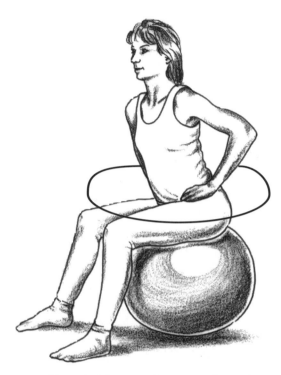

INSTRUCTION: Sit on ball in neutral position. Begin drawing a circle, initiating movement from the hips. Rotate the hips clockwise _____ time(s). Rotate the hips counter-clockwise _____ time(s).

Frequency: _____ x/day.

SPECIAL PROTOCOLS/NOTES: _Avoid making oblong circles._ _____

_____

_____

PATIENT NAME: _____ DATE: _____

THERAPIST NAME: _____

Figure Eight Pelvic Rotations

PURPOSE: To increase back and hip flexibility, and encourage motor planning.

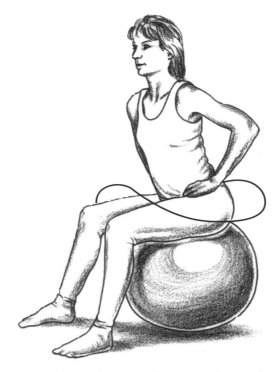

INSTRUCTION: Sit on ball in neutral position. Draw a figure "8," initiating movement from the hips. Draw the figure "8" clockwise _____ time(s). Draw the figure "8" counter-clockwise _____ time(s).

Frequency: _____ x/day.

SPECIAL PROTOCOLS/NOTES: _____

_____

_____

PATIENT NAME: _____ DATE: _____

THERAPIST NAME: _____

Trunk Flexion

PURPOSE: To strengthen back, legs, and neck muscles. To encourage proper weight shift from sitting to standing.

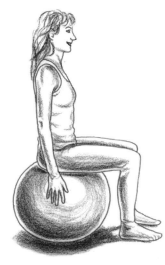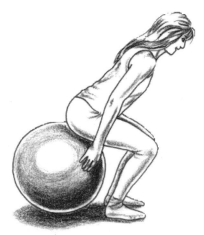

INSTRUCTION: Sit on ball in neutral position. Lean torso forward over knees.

Hold: _____ second(s).   Repeat: _____ time(s).

Frequency: _____ x/day.

SPECIAL PROTOCOLS/NOTES: _Do not lift buttocks off ball. Do not_
arch or round back.
_____
_____

PATIENT NAME: _____DATE:_____

THERAPIST NAME:_____

Shoulder Shrugs

PURPOSE: To relax shoulder muscles.

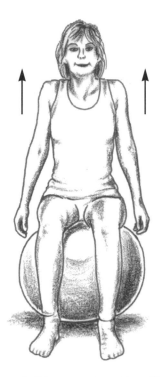

INSTRUCTION: Sit on ball in neutral position. Shrug shoulders.

Hold: _____ second(s).   Repeat: _____ time(s).

Frequency: _____ x/day.

SPECIAL PROTOCOLS/NOTES: _____

_____

_____

PATIENT NAME: _____ DATE:_____

THERAPIST NAME:_____

Bouncing on Ball Using Shoulder Shrugs

PURPOSE: To relax shoulder muscles and increase nutrition to discs in spine.

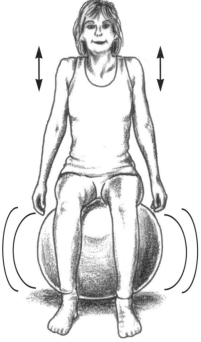

INSTRUCTION: Sit on ball in neutral position. Shrug shoulders. Repeat rhythmically to bounce ball.

Hold: _____ second(s).   Repeat: _____ time(s).

Frequency: _____ x/day.

SPECIAL PROTOCOLS/NOTES: _____

_____

_____

PATIENT NAME: _____ DATE:_____

THERAPIST NAME:_____

Shoulder Circles

PURPOSE: To relax shoulder muscles. To encourage good posture.

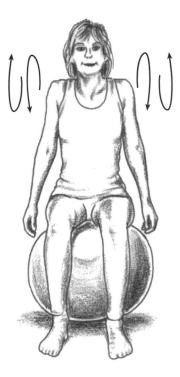

INSTRUCTION: Sit on ball in neutral position.
Gently roll shoulders backward.   Repeat _____ time(s).
Gently roll shoulders forward.   Repeat _____ time(s).

Frequency: _____ x/day.

SPECIAL PROTOCOLS/NOTES: _____

_____

_____

PATIENT NAME: _____ DATE: _____

THERAPIST NAME: _____

Arm Circles Forward

PURPOSE: To strengthen arm and upper back muscles.

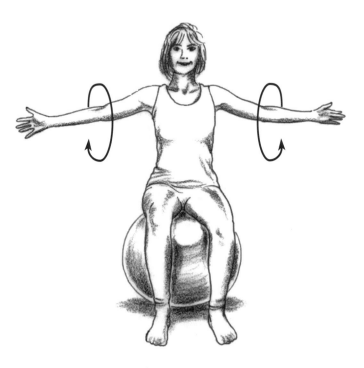

INSTRUCTION: Sit on ball in neutral position. Lift arms out away from body with thumbs up. Rotate arms forward.

Repeat: _____ time(s).   Frequency: _____ x/day.

SPECIAL PROTOCOLS/NOTES: _____

_____

_____

PATIENT NAME: _____ DATE:_____

THERAPIST NAME:_____

Arm Circles Backward

PURPOSE: To strengthen arm and upper back muscles.

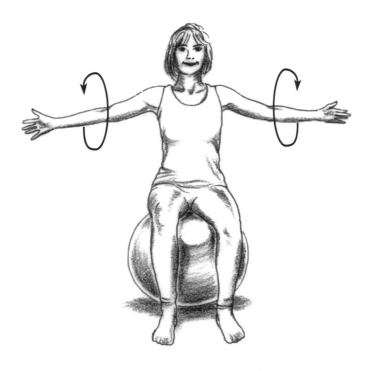

INSTRUCTION: Sit on ball in neutral position. Lift arms out away from body with thumbs up. Rotate arms backward.

Repeat: _____ time(s).   Frequency: _____ x/day.

SPECIAL PROTOCOLS/NOTES: _____

_____

_____

PATIENT NAME: _____DATE:_____

THERAPIST NAME:_____

Ball Squeeze

PURPOSE: To strengthen arm and shoulder muscles.

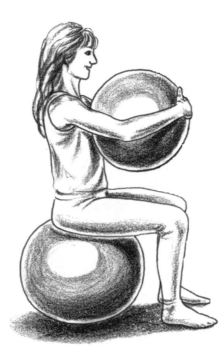

INSTRUCTION: Sit on ball in neutral position. Place second ball in arms. Hug ball and gently squeeze ball with arms.

Hold: _____ second(s).   Repeat: _____ time(s).

Frequency: _____ x/day.

SPECIAL PROTOCOLS/NOTES: _____

_____

_____

PATIENT NAME: _____ DATE:_____

THERAPIST NAME:_____

Jumping Jack

PURPOSE: To increase range of motion and strengthen shoulder muscles.

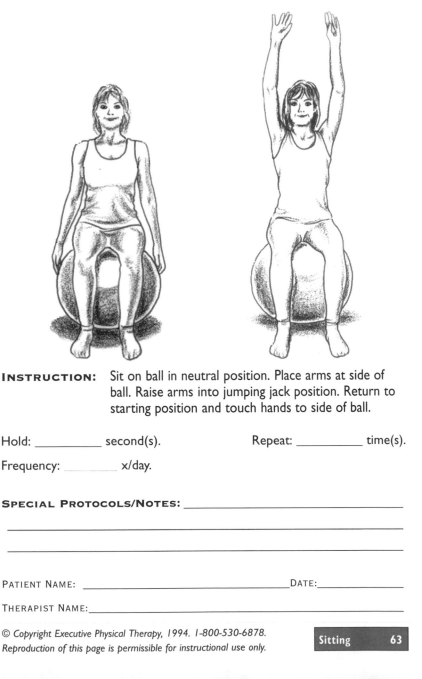

INSTRUCTION: Sit on ball in neutral position. Place arms at side of ball. Raise arms into jumping jack position. Return to starting position and touch hands to side of ball.

Hold: _____ second(s).   Repeat: _____ time(s).

Frequency: _____ x/day.

SPECIAL PROTOCOLS/NOTES: _____

_____

_____

PATIENT NAME: _____DATE:_____

THERAPIST NAME:_____

Jumping Jack with Bounce

PURPOSE: To increase range of motion and strengthen shoulder muscles. To improve coordination.

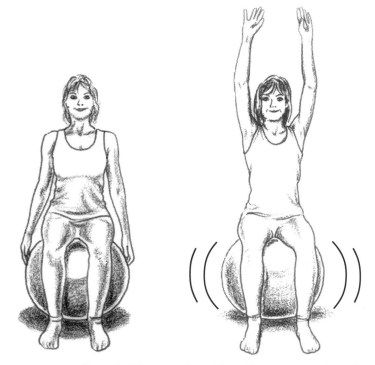

INSTRUCTION: Sit on ball in neutral position. Place arms at side of ball. Raise arms into jumping jack position. Bounce. Return to starting position and touch hands to side of ball. Bounce.

Repeat: _____ time(s).   Frequency: _____ x/day.

SPECIAL PROTOCOLS/NOTES: _____

_____

_____

PATIENT NAME: _____ DATE:_____

THERAPIST NAME:_____

The Drummer

PURPOSE: To strengthen arm, back, and neck muscles.

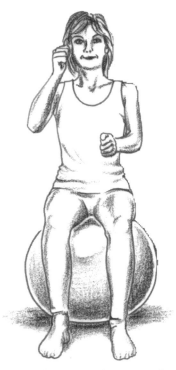

INSTRUCTION: Sit on ball in neutral position. Bend elbows. Alternate raising and lowering hands as if beating on a drum.

Hold: _____ second(s).   Repeat: _____ time(s).

Frequency: _____ x/day.

SPECIAL PROTOCOLS/NOTES: _____

_____

_____

PATIENT NAME: _____ DATE: _____

THERAPIST NAME: _____

Pronation/Supination of Hands

PURPOSE: To strengthen neck muscles. To increase range of motion in forearms.

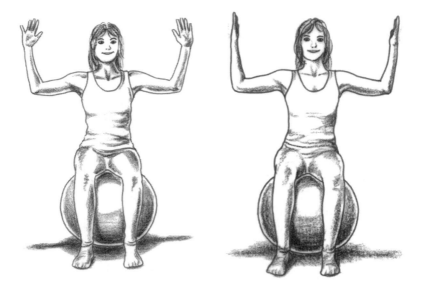

INSTRUCTION: Sit on ball in neutral position. Lift arms with elbows bent as shown. Rotate hands in and out.

Hold: _____ second(s).   Repeat: _____ time(s).

Frequency: _____ x/day.

SPECIAL PROTOCOLS/NOTES: _____

_____

_____

PATIENT NAME: _____DATE:_____

THERAPIST NAME:_____

Unilateral Shoulder Flexion

PURPOSE: To strengthen arm, back, and neck muscles.

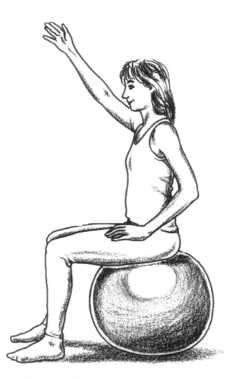

INSTRUCTION: Sit on ball in neutral position. Raise arm straight overhead and lower. Repeat with opposite arm.

Hold: _____ second(s).   Repeat: _____ time(s).

Frequency: _____ x/day.

SPECIAL PROTOCOLS/NOTES: _____

_____

_____

PATIENT NAME: _____ DATE: _____

THERAPIST NAME: _____

Reciprocal Shoulder Flexion/Extension

PURPOSE: To strengthen arm, back, and neck muscles. To improve coordination.

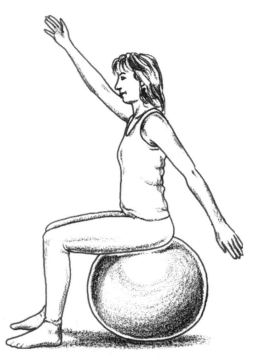

INSTRUCTION: Sit on ball in neutral position. Lift one arm in front of body and one arm behind. Keep both arms straightened. Alternate swinging arms back and forth in a gentle, rhythmic pattern.

Repeat: _____ time(s).   Frequency: _____ x/day.

SPECIAL PROTOCOLS/NOTES: _____

_____

_____

PATIENT NAME: _____DATE:_____

THERAPIST NAME:_____

Unilateral Shoulder Flexion/ Extension with a Bounce

PURPOSE: To strengthen arm, back, and neck muscles. To improve coordination.

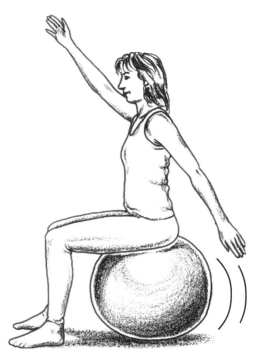

INSTRUCTION: Sit on ball in neutral position. Extend one arm in front of body and one arm behind. Keep both arms straightened. Alternate swinging arms back and forth in a gentle, rhythmic pattern. Bounce on ball as arms swing forward.

Repeat: _____ time(s).   Frequency: _____ x/day.

SPECIAL PROTOCOLS/NOTES: _____

_____

_____

PATIENT NAME: _____DATE:_____

THERAPIST NAME:_____

Contralateral Shoulder Flexion with Knee Flexion

PURPOSE: To strengthen arm and leg muscles. To improve coordination.

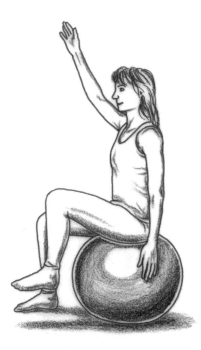

INSTRUCTION: Sit on ball. Raise right arm and left knee. Lower. Repeat with opposite arm and leg.

Hold: _____ second(s).   Repeat: _____ time(s).

Frequency: _____ x/day.

SPECIAL PROTOCOLS/NOTES: _____

_____

_____

PATIENT NAME: _____ DATE: _____

THERAPIST NAME: _____

Ipsilateral Shoulder Flexion
and Hip Flexion

PURPOSE: To strengthen arm and leg muscles. To improve balance
reactions.

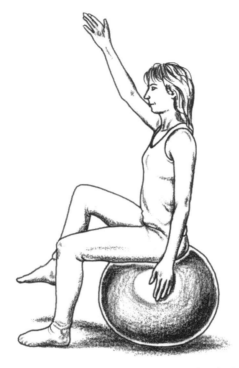

INSTRUCTION: Sit on ball. Raise right arm and right knee. Lower.
Repeat with opposite side.

Hold: _____ second(s).   Repeat: _____ time(s).

Frequency: _____ x/day.

SPECIAL PROTOCOLS/NOTES: _____

_____

_____

PATIENT NAME: _____DATE:_____

THERAPIST NAME:_____

Marching in Seated Position

PURPOSE: To strengthen leg muscles. To improve balance and coordination.

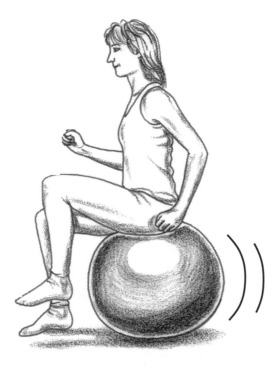

INSTRUCTION: Sit on ball in neutral position. March in a rhythmic pattern.

Repeat: _____ time(s).   Frequency: _____ x/day.

SPECIAL PROTOCOLS/NOTES: _Arm should swing with opposite leg._

_____

_____

PATIENT NAME: _____DATE:_____

THERAPIST NAME:_____

Trunk Rotation

PURPOSE: To strengthen arm muscles. To increase trunk flexibility.

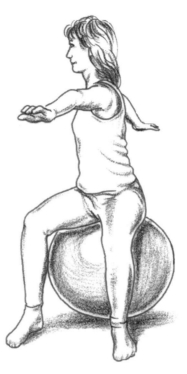

INSTRUCTION: Sit on ball. Extend arms and rotate. Repeat to other side.

Hold: _____ second(s).   Repeat: _____ time(s).

Frequency: _____ x/day.

SPECIAL PROTOCOLS/NOTES: _____

_____

_____

PATIENT NAME: _____ DATE: _____

THERAPIST NAME: _____

Trunk Rotation
with Small Ball

PURPOSE: To increase trunk flexibility. To strengthen abdominal and arm muscles.

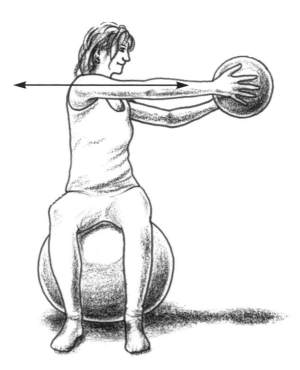

INSTRUCTION: Sit on ball. Grasp small ball between hands. Straighten arms and raise to shoulder height. Rotate arms to the left and then to the right. Watch ball throughout motion.

Hold: _____ second(s).   Repeat: _____ time(s).

Frequency: _____ x/day.

SPECIAL PROTOCOLS/NOTES: _____

_____

_____

PATIENT NAME: _____DATE:_____

THERAPIST NAME:_____

Trunk Diagonal Rotation
with Small Ball

PURPOSE: To increase trunk flexibility. To strengthen arm and oblique abdominal muscles.

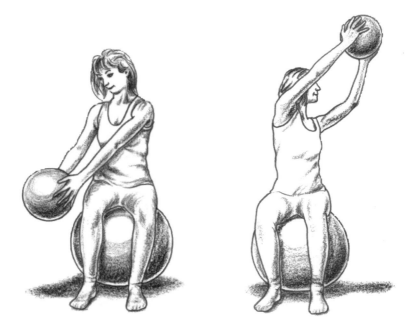

INSTRUCTION: Sit on ball. Grasp small ball between hands. Straighten arms and place near outside of right thigh. Raise arms over left shoulder. Watch ball and rotate head throughout motion. Repeat with opposite side.

Hold: _____ second(s).   Repeat: _____ time(s).

Frequency: _____ x/day.

SPECIAL PROTOCOLS/NOTES: _____

_____

_____

PATIENT NAME: _____ **DATE:** _____

THERAPIST NAME: _____

Ball Overhead

PURPOSE: To strengthen arm, back, and neck muscles.

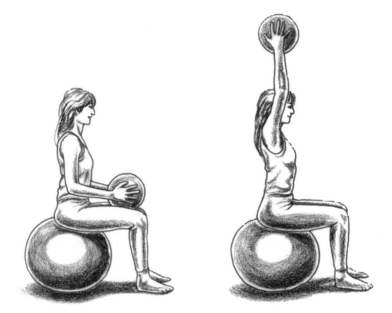

INSTRUCTION: Sit on ball in neutral position. Place small ball in hands. Raise hands overhead. Straighten arms.

Hold: _____ second(s).   Repeat: _____ time(s).

Frequency: _____ x/day.

SPECIAL PROTOCOLS/NOTES: Do not arch back. _____

_____

_____

PATIENT NAME: _____ DATE: _____

THERAPIST NAME: _____

Ball from Knees to Toes

PURPOSE: To stretch back and upper body muscles.

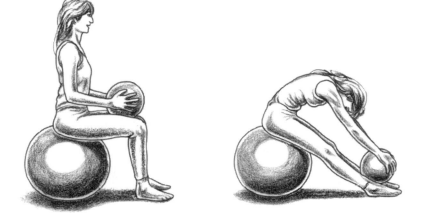

INSTRUCTION: Sit on ball. Place small ball in hands. Push large ball back with buttocks and extend legs. Roll small ball down legs.

Hold: _____ second(s).   Repeat: _____ time(s).

Frequency: _____ x/day.

SPECIAL PROTOCOLS/NOTES: _____

_____

_____

PATIENT NAME: _____ DATE: _____

THERAPIST NAME: _____

Ball Overhead to Knees to Toes

PURPOSE: To strengthen arm, back, and neck muscles. To stretch back and upper body.

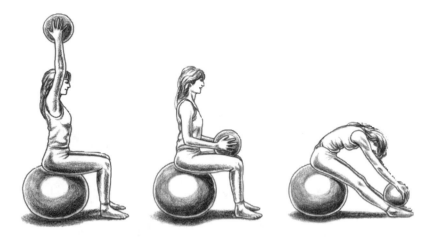

INSTRUCTION: Sit on ball in neutral position. Place small ball in hands. Raise arms overhead. Lower hands to knees. Push large ball back with buttocks and extend legs. Roll second ball down legs.

Hold: _____ second(s).   Repeat: _____ time(s).

Frequency: _____ x/day.

SPECIAL PROTOCOLS/NOTES: _____

_____

_____

PATIENT NAME: _____ DATE:_____

THERAPIST NAME:_____

Sit Back

PURPOSE: To strengthen abdominal muscles.

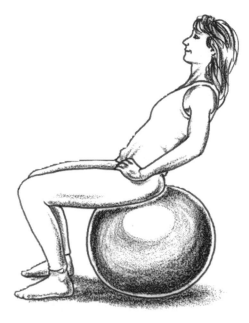

INSTRUCTION: Sit on ball. Recline backward on ball. Keep head and chin up. Hold _____ second(s). Return to upright position.

Repeat: _____ time(s).   Frequency: _____ x/day.

SPECIAL PROTOCOLS/NOTES: _Do not arch back. Do not bend at_ waist.

_____

PATIENT NAME: _____ DATE: _____

THERAPIST NAME: _____

Crossing Arms

PURPOSE: To strengthen oblique abdominal muscles.

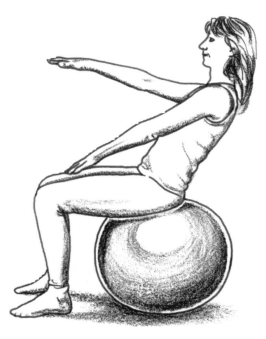

INSTRUCTION: Sit on ball. Recline backward on ball. Extend arms in front of body. Touch right knee with left hand. Hold _____ second(s). Repeat with opposite hand.

Repeat: _____ time(s).   Frequency: _____ x/day.

SPECIAL PROTOCOLS/NOTES: ___Keep chin up. Do not arch back.___

_____

_____

PATIENT NAME: _____DATE:_____

THERAPIST NAME:_____

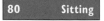

Abdominal Oblique Sit Back

Purpose: To strengthen oblique abdominal muscles.

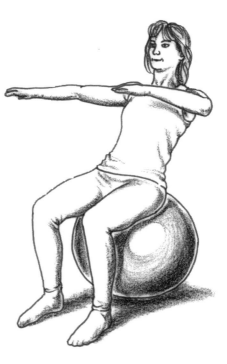

Instruction: Sit on ball. Lean backward on ball. Extend right arm out to side of body. Touch left hand to right shoulder. Hold _____ second(s). Repeat on opposite side.

Repeat: _____ time(s).   Frequency: _____ x/day.

Special Protocols/Notes: ___Do not bend at waist. Do not arch___ back._____

_____

Patient Name: _____Date:_____

Therapist Name:_____

Cross Arms to Overhead

PURPOSE: To strengthen abdominal, arm, and neck muscles.

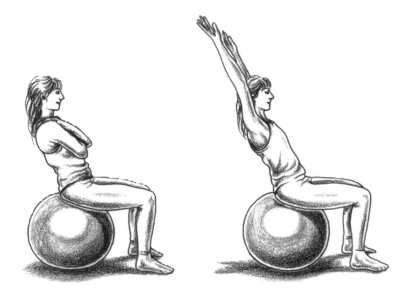

INSTRUCTION: Sit on ball in neutral position. Cross arms across chest. Lean back slightly and extend arms overhead.

Hold: _____ second(s).   Repeat: _____ time(s).

Frequency: _____ x/day.

SPECIAL PROTOCOLS/NOTES: _____

_____

_____

PATIENT NAME: _____DATE:_____

THERAPIST NAME:_____

Diagonal Arm Lifts

PURPOSE: To strengthen oblique abdominal, arm, back, and neck muscles.

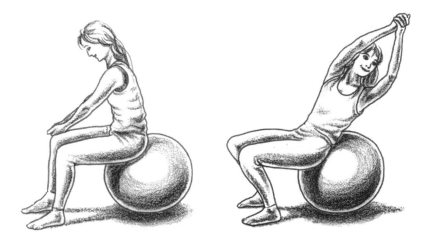

INSTRUCTION: Sit on ball. Clasp hands and place by right knee. Roll ball forward while leaning backward. Raise hands over left shoulder. Watch hands throughout motion. Repeat with hands by left knee, raising over right shoulder.

Hold: _____ second(s).   Repeat: _____ time(s).

Frequency: _____ x/day.

SPECIAL PROTOCOLS/NOTES: _____

_____

_____

PATIENT NAME: _____DATE:_____

THERAPIST NAME:_____

Full Sit Back

PURPOSE: To strengthen abdominal and neck muscles.

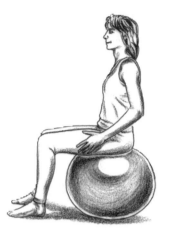

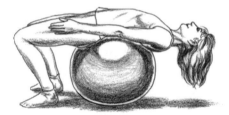

INSTRUCTION: Sit on ball in neutral position. Lean backward as ball is rolled forward with hips. Return to starting position.

Repeat: _____ time(s).   Frequency: _____ x/day.

SPECIAL PROTOCOLS/NOTES: Do not bend at waist. Keep distance between chin and navel the same when going from sitting position to full sit back position.

PATIENT NAME: _____ DATE:_____

THERAPIST NAME:_____

Heel Raises

PURPOSE: To strengthen ankle and leg muscles. To increase range of motion in ankles.

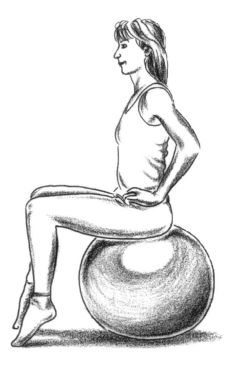

INSTRUCTION: Sit on ball. Raise heels off floor. Lower heels to floor.

Hold: _____ second(s).   Repeat: _____ time(s).

Frequency: _____ x/day.

SPECIAL PROTOCOLS/NOTES: _____

_____

_____

PATIENT NAME: _____ DATE:_____

THERAPIST NAME:_____

Eccentric Contraction
of Calf Muscles

PURPOSE: To increase strength and coordination in ankle and leg muscles.

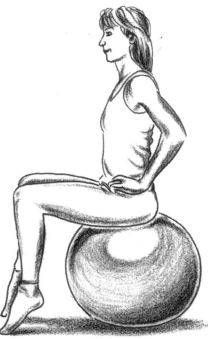

INSTRUCTION: Sit on ball. Raise heels off floor. Rapidly lower heels, however, do not touch floor. Repeat in a rapid, rhythmic pattern.

Repeat: _____ time(s).   Frequency: _____ x/day.

SPECIAL PROTOCOLS/NOTES: _____

_____

_____

PATIENT NAME: _____ DATE: _____

THERAPIST NAME: _____

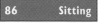

Toe Raises

PURPOSE: To increase strength and coordination in ankle and leg muscles.

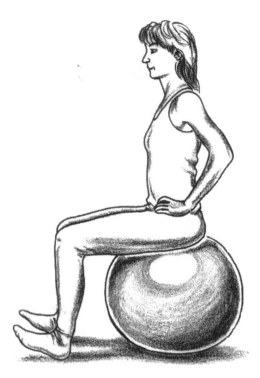

INSTRUCTION: Sit on ball in neutral position. Tap toes to floor.

Hold: _____ second(s).   Repeat: _____ time(s).

Frequency: _____ x/day.

SPECIAL PROTOCOLS/NOTES: _____

_____

_____

PATIENT NAME: _____ DATE:_____

THERAPIST NAME:_____

Eccentric Contraction
of Anterior Lower Leg

PURPOSE: To increase strength and coordination in ankle and leg muscles.

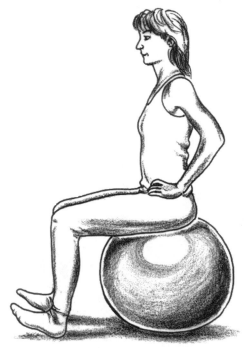

INSTRUCTION: Sit on ball in neutral position. Raise toes upward. Rapidly lower toes, but do not touch toes to floor. Repeat rapidly in a rhythmic pattern.

Repeat: _____ time(s).   Frequency: _____ x/day.

SPECIAL PROTOCOLS/NOTES: _____

_____

_____

PATIENT NAME: _____DATE:_____

THERAPIST NAME:_____

Toe Flick with Mini Ball

PURPOSE: To increase range of motion and strength in toes.

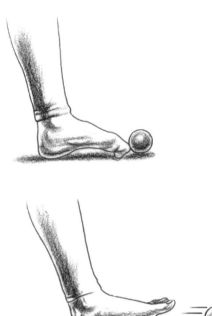

INSTRUCTION: Sit in chair. Curl toes under. Place mini ball in front of toes. Flick ball with toes. Repeat with opposite side.

Hold: _____ second(s).   Repeat: _____ time(s).

Frequency: _____ x/day.

SPECIAL PROTOCOLS/NOTES: _____

_____

_____

PATIENT NAME: _____ DATE:_____

THERAPIST NAME:_____

Knee Flexion/Extension
with Mini Ball

PURPOSE: To strengthen ankle and leg muscles.

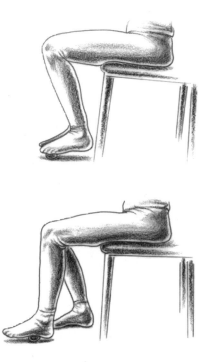

INSTRUCTION: Sit on chair. Bend knee and place mini ball under toes. Straighten knee until ball rolls to heel. Roll ball back and forth between toes and heel in a rapid, rhythmic pattern. Repeat with opposite side.

Repeat: _____ time(s).   Frequency: _____ x/day.

SPECIAL PROTOCOLS/NOTES: _____

_____

_____

PATIENT NAME: _____DATE:_____

THERAPIST NAME:_____

Knee Flexion/Extension with Small Ball

PURPOSE: To increase range of motion and strength in knee and leg muscles.

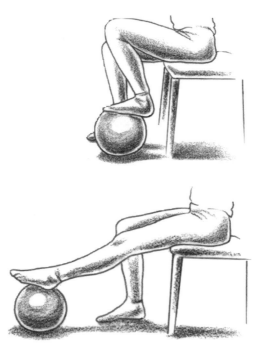

INSTRUCTION: Sit on chair. Bend knee and place ball under foot. Straighten knee. Repeat with opposite side.

Hold: _____ second(s).   Repeat: _____ time(s).

Frequency: _____ x/day.

SPECIAL PROTOCOLS/NOTES: _____

_____

_____

PATIENT NAME: _____ DATE: _____

THERAPIST NAME: _____

Knee Extension

PURPOSE: To strengthen knee and leg muscles.

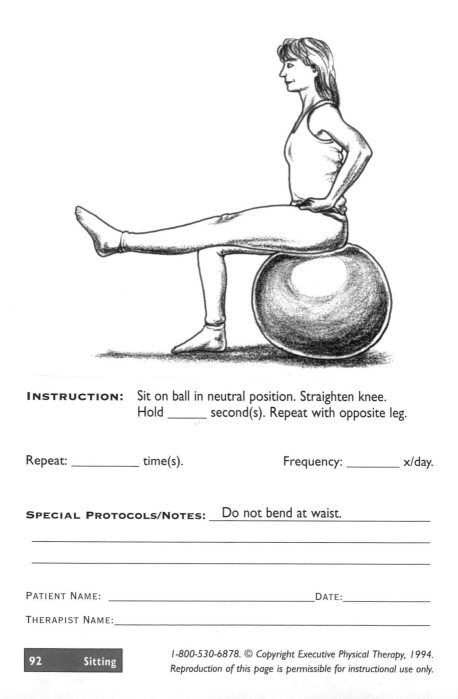

INSTRUCTION: Sit on ball in neutral position. Straighten knee.
Hold _____ second(s). Repeat with opposite leg.

Repeat: _____ time(s).   Frequency: _____ x/day.

SPECIAL PROTOCOLS/NOTES: __Do not bend at waist._____

_____

_____

PATIENT NAME: _____DATE:_____

THERAPIST NAME:_____

Write Alphabet with Foot

PURPOSE: To strengthen ankle, knee, and leg muscles. To improve balance reactions.

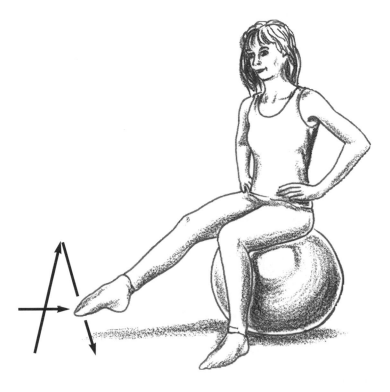

INSTRUCTION: Sit on ball in neutral position. Straighten knee. Write alphabet with foot. Repeat with opposite side.

Repeat: _____ time(s).   Frequency: _____ x/day.

SPECIAL PROTOCOLS/NOTES: __Do not slouch._____

_____

_____

PATIENT NAME: _____ DATE:_____

THERAPIST NAME:_____

Knee Adduction Squeeze

PURPOSE: To strengthen knee muscles.

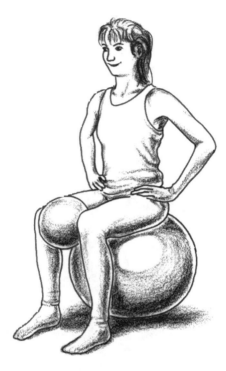

INSTRUCTION: Sit on large ball. Place smaller ball between knees.
Squeeze ball with knees.

Hold: _____ second(s).   Repeat: _____ time(s).

Frequency: _____ x/day.

SPECIAL PROTOCOLS/NOTES: _____

_____

_____

PATIENT NAME: _____DATE:_____

THERAPIST NAME:_____

Hip Internal/External Rotation with Mini Ball

PURPOSE: To increase range of motion and strengthen ankle, hip, and leg muscles.

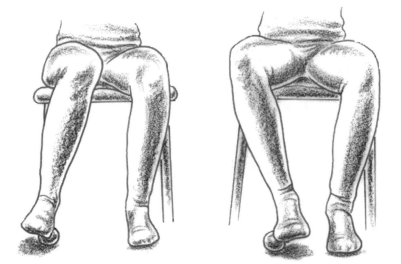

INSTRUCTION: Sit on chair. Bend knee and place mini ball under toes. Roll ball to inside and outside of foot in a rapid, rhythmic pattern. Repeat with opposite foot.

Repeat: _____ time(s).   Frequency: _____ x/day.

SPECIAL PROTOCOLS/NOTES: _Allow knee to move in the opposite_ direction of the foot. _____

_____

PATIENT NAME: _____ DATE: _____

THERAPIST NAME: _____

Hip Internal/External Rotation with Small Ball

PURPOSE: To increase range of motion and strength in hips.

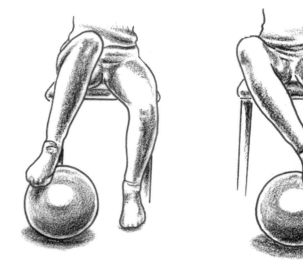

INSTRUCTION: Sit on chair. Lift knee and place small ball under foot. Roll ball from side to side with foot. Repeat with opposite foot.

Hold: _____ second(s).   Repeat: _____ time(s).

Frequency: _____ x/day.

SPECIAL PROTOCOLS/NOTES: _Allow knee to move in the opposite_
direction of the foot. _____

_____

PATIENT NAME: _____DATE:_____

THERAPIST NAME:_____

Hip Internal/External Rotation

PURPOSE: To increase range of motion and strength in hips.

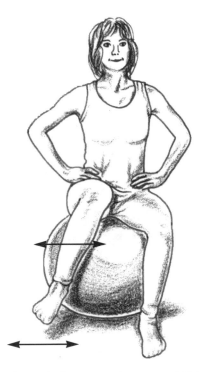

INSTRUCTION: Sit on ball in neutral position. Lift knee and turn foot in and out. Repeat with opposite side.

Hold: _____ second(s).   Repeat: _____ time(s).

Frequency: _____ x/day.

SPECIAL PROTOCOLS/NOTES: _____

_____

_____

PATIENT NAME: _____DATE:_____

THERAPIST NAME:_____

Unilateral Hip Flexion

PURPOSE: To strengthen hip and leg muscles. To challenge balance reactions.

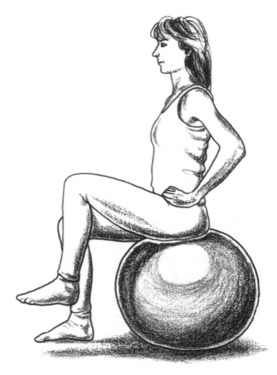

INSTRUCTION: Sit on ball in neutral position. Raise knee.
Hold _____ second(s). Repeat with opposite knee.

Repeat: _____ time(s).   Frequency: _____ x/day.

SPECIAL PROTOCOLS/NOTES: _____

_____

_____

PATIENT NAME: _____ DATE:_____

THERAPIST NAME:_____

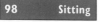

Unilateral Hip Flexion with Bounce

PURPOSE: To strengthen hip and leg muscles. To challenge balance reactions.

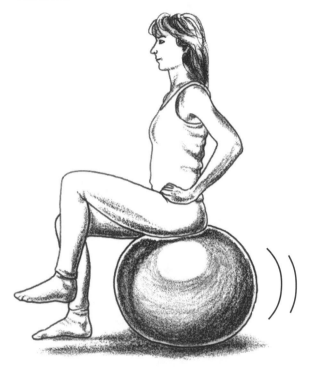

INSTRUCTION: Sit on ball in neutral position. Raise knee. Begin bouncing. Repeat with opposite knee.

Hold: _____ second(s).   Repeat: _____ time(s).

Frequency: _____ x/day.

SPECIAL PROTOCOLS/NOTES: _____

_____

_____

PATIENT NAME: _____ DATE: _____

THERAPIST NAME: _____

Balance on Ball
with Feet on Second Ball

PURPOSE: To improve balance reactions.

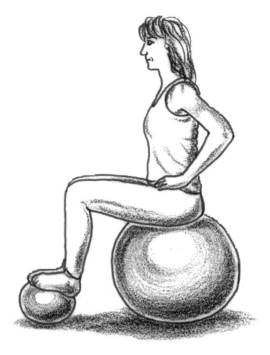

INSTRUCTION: Sit on ball. Place small ball under feet. Maintain balance and keep neutral position with back.

Hold: _____ second(s).   Repeat: _____ time(s).

Frequency: _____ x/day.

SPECIAL PROTOCOLS/NOTES: _____

_____

_____

PATIENT NAME: _____ DATE:_____

THERAPIST NAME:_____

Balance on Ball
Without Feet

PURPOSE: To strengthen abdominal, arm, and leg muscles. To improve balance reactions.

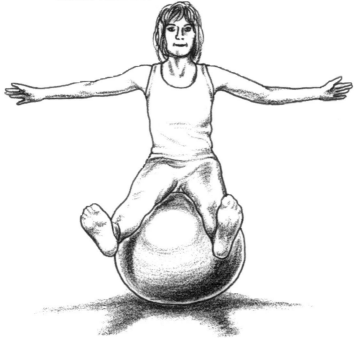

INSTRUCTION: Sit on ball in neutral position. Extend arms out to side of body. Lift and extend legs out away from ball.

Hold: _____ second(s).   Repeat: _____ time(s).

Frequency: _____ x/day.

SPECIAL PROTOCOLS/NOTES: Do not overextend legs. _____

_____

_____

PATIENT NAME: _____DATE:_____

THERAPIST NAME:_____

Shoulder and Trunk Flexion

PURPOSE: To strengthen abdominal, arm, back, and neck muscles.

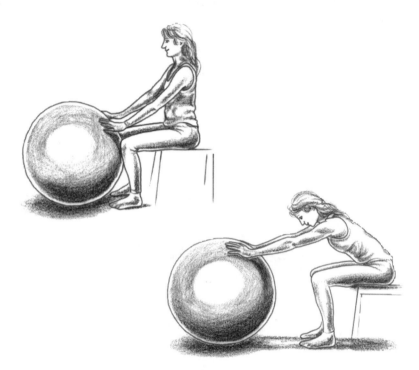

INSTRUCTION: Sit on a chair. Place hands on ball in front of body. Straighten arms. Roll ball forward with hands. Lean forward with body.

Hold: _____ second(s).   Repeat: _____ time(s).

Frequency: _____ x/day.

SPECIAL PROTOCOLS/NOTES: _____

_____

_____

PATIENT NAME: _____DATE:_____

THERAPIST NAME:_____

Shoulder Rolls

PURPOSE: To increase range of motion in shoulders and trunk. To strengthen abdominal, arm, back, and neck muscles.

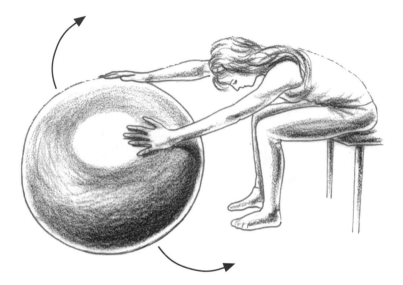

INSTRUCTION: Sit on chair. Place hands on ball in front of body. Straighten arms. Roll ball forward with hands. Lean forward with body. Roll ball from side to side with hands.

Hold: _____ second(s).   Repeat: _____ time(s).

Frequency: _____ x/day.

SPECIAL PROTOCOLS/NOTES: _____

_____

_____

PATIENT NAME: _____ DATE: _____

THERAPIST NAME: _____

Lateral Trunk Shift with Cervical Rotation

PURPOSE: To increase range of motion and strength in neck, shoulders, and trunk.

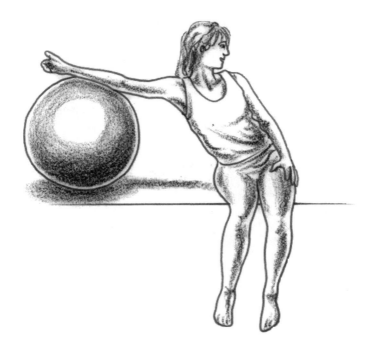

INSTRUCTION: Sit on table. Place ball under right hand and extend arm out to side of body. Turn thumb up toward ceiling. Rotate head to the left and look over shoulder. Lean to right side. Repeat with opposite side.

Hold: _____ second(s).   Repeat: _____ time(s).

Frequency: _____ x/day.

SPECIAL PROTOCOLS/NOTES: _____

_____

_____

PATIENT NAME: _____DATE:_____

THERAPIST NAME:_____

Lateral Trunk Shift

PURPOSE: To increase range of motion and strength in shoulders and trunk.

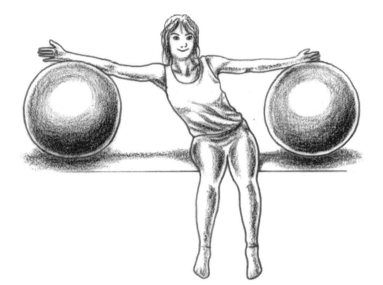

INSTRUCTION: Sit on table. Place one ball under each hand. Extend arms out to side of body. Turn thumbs up toward ceiling. Lean side to side.

Hold: _____ second(s).   Repeat: _____ time(s).

Frequency: _____ x/day.

SPECIAL PROTOCOLS/NOTES: _____

_____

_____

PATIENT NAME: _____ DATE: _____

THERAPIST NAME: _____

Bilateral Horizontal Abduction/Adduction

PURPOSE: To increase range of motion and strength in shoulders.

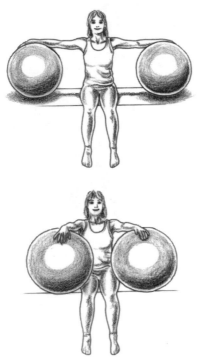

INSTRUCTION: Sit on table. Place one ball under each hand. Extend arms out to side of body. Roll balls forward to front of body.

Hold: _____ second(s). Repeat: _____ time(s).

Frequency: _____ x/day.

SPECIAL PROTOCOLS/NOTES: _____

_____

_____

PATIENT NAME: _____ DATE:_____

THERAPIST NAME:_____

Trunk Rotation

PURPOSE: To increase range of motion and strength in shoulders and trunk.

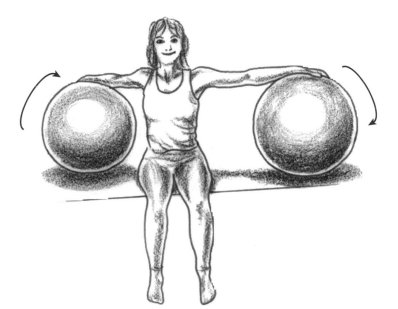

INSTRUCTION: Sit on table. Place one ball under each hand. Rotate right arm backward and left arm forward. Keep head facing forward. Repeat with opposite side.

Hold: _____ second(s).   Repeat: _____ time(s).

Frequency: _____ x/day.

SPECIAL PROTOCOLS/NOTES: _____

_____

_____

PATIENT NAME: _____DATE:_____

THERAPIST NAME:_____

Cervical and Trunk Rotation

PURPOSE: To increase range of motion and strength in neck, shoulders, and trunk.

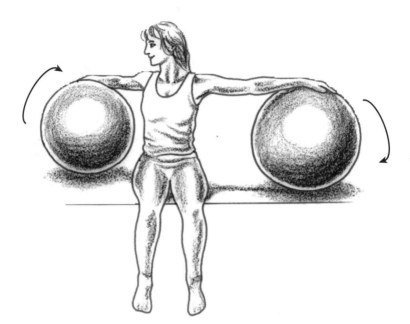

INSTRUCTION: Sit on table. Place one ball under each hand. Look over right shoulder. Rotate right arm backward and left arm forward. Repeat with opposite side.

Hold: _____ second(s).   Repeat: _____ time(s).

Frequency: _____ x/day.

SPECIAL PROTOCOLS/NOTES: _____

_____

_____

PATIENT NAME: _____ DATE: _____

THERAPIST NAME: _____

The Pike

PURPOSE: To strengthen abdominal, arm, and leg muscles.

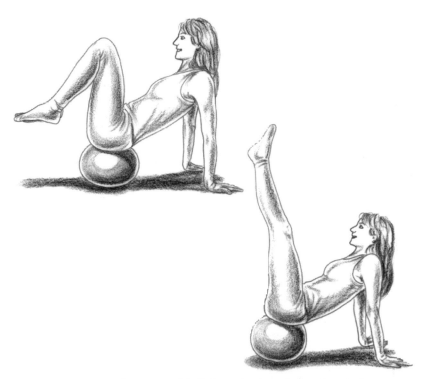

INSTRUCTION: Sit on small ball. Lean back and place hands flat on floor behind ball. Bend knees toward chest. Straighten knees and raise toes toward ceiling.

Hold: _____ second(s).   Repeat: _____ time(s).

Frequency: _____ x/day.

SPECIAL PROTOCOLS/NOTES: _____

_____

_____

PATIENT NAME: _____ DATE:_____

THERAPIST NAME:_____

Unilateral Lower Extremity Kip

PURPOSE: To strengthen abdominal, arm, and leg muscles.

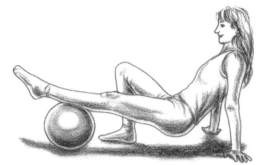

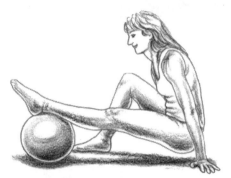

INSTRUCTION: Sit on floor. Bend one knee and place opposite foot on small ball with leg straightened. Lift hips off floor. Swing hips back toward hands as ball rolls toward foot. Repeat in a rapid, rhythmic pattern. Repeat with opposite side.

Hold: _____ second(s).   Repeat: _____ time(s).

Frequency: _____ x/day.

SPECIAL PROTOCOLS/NOTES: _____

_____

_____

PATIENT NAME: _____DATE:_____

THERAPIST NAME:_____

Lower Extremity Kip

PURPOSE: To strengthen abdominal, arm, and leg muscles.

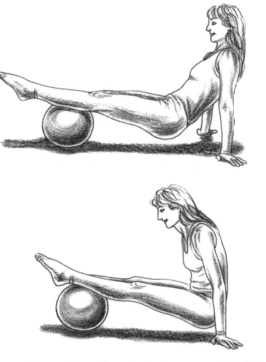

INSTRUCTION: Sit on floor. Place both feet on small ball. Straighten
legs. Place hands flat on floor behind back. Lift hips off
floor. Swing hips back toward hands as ball rolls
toward feet. Repeat in a rapid, rhythmic pattern.

Hold: _____ second(s).   Repeat: _____ time(s).

Frequency: _____ x/day.

SPECIAL PROTOCOLS/NOTES: _____

_____

_____

PATIENT NAME: _____ DATE:_____

THERAPIST NAME:_____

The Twister

PURPOSE: To strengthen abdominal, arm, and inner thigh muscles. To improve trunk flexibility.

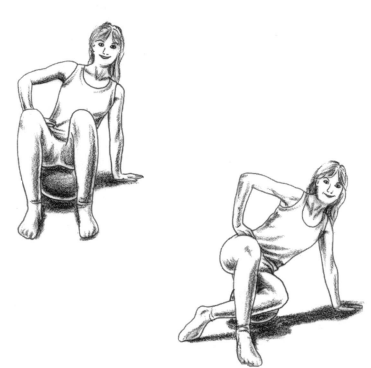

INSTRUCTION: Sit on small ball. Place right hand on hip. Lean back and place left hand flat on floor. Shift weight onto left hip as left leg moves under right knee. Return to starting position. Repeat with opposite side.

Hold: _____ second(s).   Repeat: _____ time(s).

Frequency: _____ x/day.

SPECIAL PROTOCOLS/NOTES: _____

_____

_____

PATIENT NAME: _____ DATE:_____

THERAPIST NAME:_____

CHAPTER FOUR

Supine

Neutral Position in Supine

PURPOSE: To strengthen muscles in an optimal position to avoid injury.

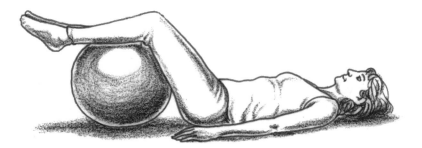

INSTRUCTION: Lie on back with legs on ball.

Hold: _____ second(s).   Repeat: ____ ____ time(s).

Frequency: _____ x/day.

SPECIAL PROTOCOLS/NOTES: Do not arch back or flatten back.
   Maintain natural curve in back. _____

_____

PATIENT NAME: _____ DATE:_____

THERAPIST NAME:_____

Knee Rolls

PURPOSE: To stretch muscles in torso.

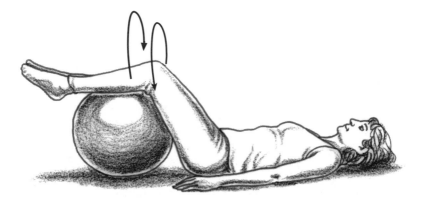

INSTRUCTION: Lie on back with legs on ball. Roll ball from side to side using knees.

Hold: _____ second(s).   Repeat: _____ time(s).

Frequency: _____ x/day.

SPECIAL PROTOCOLS/NOTES: Do not lift shoulders off floor. _____

_____

_____

PATIENT NAME: _____DATE:_____

THERAPIST NAME:_____

Trunk Counter Rotation
with Knees on Ball

PURPOSE: To strengthen oblique abdominal muscles. To stretch muscles
in trunk. To improve coordination of upper and lower body.

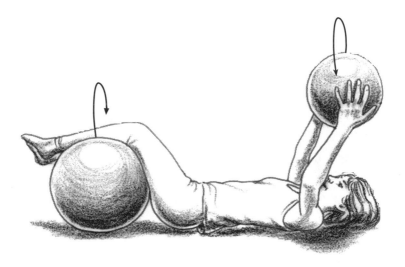

INSTRUCTION: Lie on back. Rest knees on top of ball. Place a small
ball between hands and raise arms. Move arms to left
and knees to right. Repeat in opposite direction.

Hold: _____ second(s).   Repeat: _____ time(s).

Frequency: _____ x/day.

SPECIAL PROTOCOLS/NOTES: _____

_____

_____

PATIENT NAME: _____ DATE:_____

THERAPIST NAME:_____

Trunk Counter Rotation

PURPOSE: To stretch muscles in trunk. To improve coordination of upper and lower body.

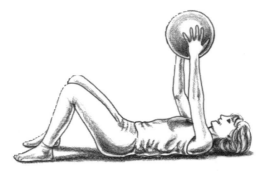

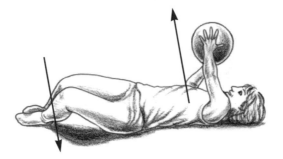

INSTRUCTION: Lie on back and bend knees. Place small ball between hands and raise arms. Move arms to right and knees to left. Repeat in opposite direction.

Hold: _____ second(s).   Repeat: _____ time(s).

Frequency: _____ x/day.

SPECIAL PROTOCOLS/NOTES: _____

_____

_____

PATIENT NAME: _____DATE:_____

THERAPIST NAME:_____

Supine Shoulder Abduction/Adduction

PURPOSE: To increase range of motion and strengthen shoulder muscles.

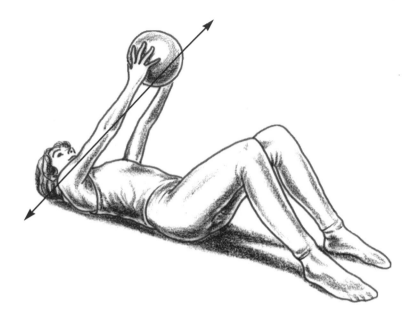

INSTRUCTION: Lie on back. Bend knees. Place small ball between hands. Extend arms. Move ball from side to side. Reach as far as arms can stretch.

Hold: _____ second(s).   Repeat: _____ time(s).

Frequency: _____ x/day.

SPECIAL PROTOCOLS/NOTES: _____

_____

_____

PATIENT NAME: _____ DATE: _____

THERAPIST NAME: _____

Bilateral Elbow Flexion/Extension

PURPOSE: To strengthen arm muscles.

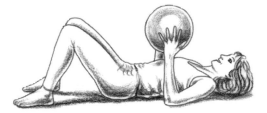

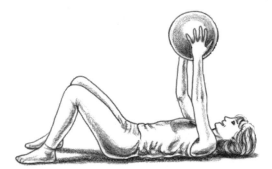

INSTRUCTION: Lie on back and bend knees. Place small ball between hands. Raise arms toward ceiling.

Hold: _____ second(s).   Repeat: _____ time(s).

Frequency: _____ x/day.

SPECIAL PROTOCOLS/NOTES: _____

_____

_____

PATIENT NAME: _____ DATE:_____

THERAPIST NAME:_____

Shoulder Internal/External Rotation

PURPOSE: To increase range of motion and strengthen shoulder muscles.

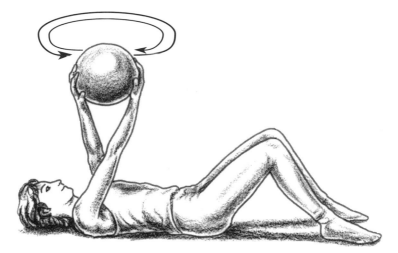

INSTRUCTION: Lie on back. Bend knees. Place small ball between hands and extend arms. Rotate ball clockwise and counter-clockwise.

Repeat: _____ time(s).   Frequency: _____ x/day.

SPECIAL PROTOCOLS/NOTES: _____

_____

_____

PATIENT NAME: _____DATE:_____

THERAPIST NAME:_____

Hip Extension with Ball under Knees

PURPOSE: To strengthen back of leg and buttock muscles.

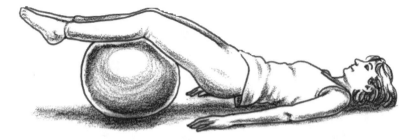

INSTRUCTION: Lie on back with legs on ball. Lift hips off floor.

Hold: _____ second(s).   Repeat: _____ time(s).

Frequency: _____ x/day.

SPECIAL PROTOCOLS/NOTES: _____

_____

_____

PATIENT NAME: _____ DATE: _____

THERAPIST NAME: _____

Abdominal Curl with Hip Extension

PURPOSE: To strengthen abdominal, back of leg, and buttock muscles.

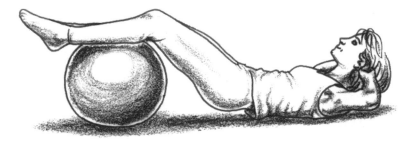

INSTRUCTION: Lie on back with legs on ball. Lift hips off floor. Place unclasped hands behind head. Raise head off floor.

Hold: _____ second(s).   Repeat: _____ time(s).

Frequency: _____ x/day.

SPECIAL PROTOCOLS/NOTES: ___Do not pull head up with hands.___

_____

_____

PATIENT NAME: _____ DATE: _____

THERAPIST NAME: _____

Supine   123

Hip Extension
with Feet on Ball

PURPOSE: To increase range of motion in hips. To strengthen leg and buttock muscles.

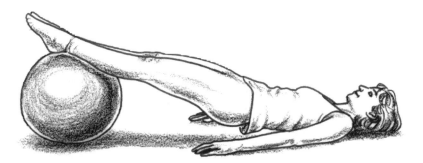

INSTRUCTION: Lie on back with feet on ball. Lift hips off floor. Keep legs straight.

Hold: _____ second(s).   Repeat: _____ time(s).

Frequency: _____ x/day.

SPECIAL PROTOCOLS/NOTES: _____

_____

_____

PATIENT NAME: _____ DATE: _____

THERAPIST NAME: _____

Leg Rolls

PURPOSE: To strengthen hip, leg, and oblique abdominal muscles.

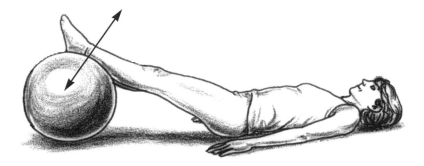

INSTRUCTION: Lie on back with heels resting on ball. Roll ball from side to side with feet. Keep legs straight.

Hold: _____ second(s). Repeat: _____ time(s).

Frequency: _____ x/day.

SPECIAL PROTOCOLS/NOTES: _____

_____

_____

PATIENT NAME: _____ DATE: _____

THERAPIST NAME: _____

Supine   125

Hip Extension
with Feet Crossed

PURPOSE: To strengthen leg and back muscles. To improve balance reactions.

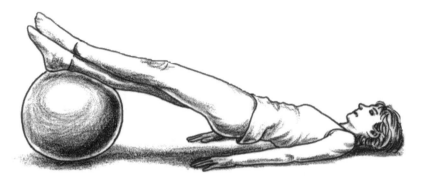

INSTRUCTION: Lie on back with heels on ball. Cross feet and raise hips off floor. Keep legs straight.

Hold: _____ second(s).   Repeat: _____ time(s).

Frequency: _____ x/day.

SPECIAL PROTOCOLS/NOTES: _____

_____

_____

PATIENT NAME: _____ DATE: _____

THERAPIST NAME: _____

Unilateral Straight Leg Raise with Hip Extension

PURPOSE: To increase strength in back, hip, and leg muscles. To improve balance reactions.

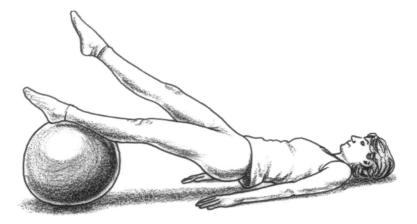

INSTRUCTION: Lie on back with both heels on ball. Lift hips off floor. Raise one leg toward ceiling. Keep legs straight. Repeat with other leg.

Hold: _____ second(s).   Repeat: _____ time(s).

Frequency: _____ x/day.

SPECIAL PROTOCOLS/NOTES: Do not arch back. _____

_____

_____

PATIENT NAME: _____DATE:_____

THERAPIST NAME:_____

Write Alphabet with Foot in Hip Extension

PURPOSE: To strengthen ankle, buttock, and leg muscles. To improve balance reactions.

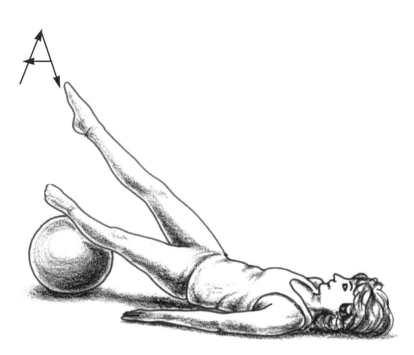

INSTRUCTION: Lie on back. Extend legs and place ball under feet. Lift hips off floor. Lift one leg off ball and begin writing alphabet with foot. Keep legs straight. Repeat with opposite leg.

Hold: _____ second(s).   Repeat: _____ time(s).

Frequency: _____ x/day.

SPECIAL PROTOCOLS/NOTES: _____

_____

_____

PATIENT NAME: _____DATE:_____

THERAPIST NAME:_____

Knee Flexion
with Hip Extension

PURPOSE: To strengthen back, hip, and leg muscles.

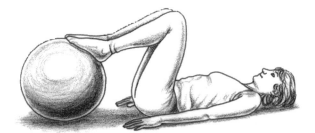

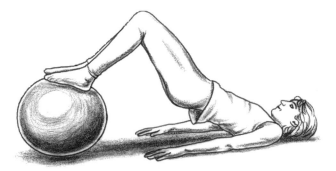

INSTRUCTION: Lie on back with knees bent and feet on ball. Lift hips off floor.

Hold: _____ second(s).   Repeat: _____ time(s).

Frequency: _____ x/day.

SPECIAL PROTOCOLS/NOTES: _____

_____

_____

PATIENT NAME: _____ DATE:_____

THERAPIST NAME:_____

Knee Flexion to Knee Extension in Hip Extension

PURPOSE: To strengthen back, hip, leg, neck, and shoulder muscles. To improve balance reactions.

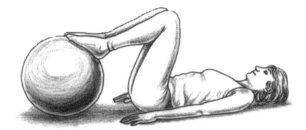

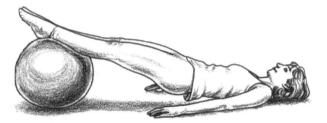

INSTRUCTION: Lie on back with knees bent and feet on ball. Lift hips off floor. Straighten knees.

Hold: _____ second(s).   Repeat: _____ time(s).

Frequency: _____ x/day.

SPECIAL PROTOCOLS/NOTES: _____

_____

_____

PATIENT NAME: _____ DATE:_____

THERAPIST NAME:_____

Short Arc Quad

PURPOSE: To increase range of motion and strengthen knee and leg muscles.

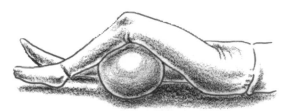

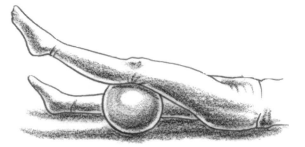

INSTRUCTION: Lie on back. Bend knee and place small ball under knee. Straighten knee. Repeat with opposite knee.

Hold: _____ second(s).   Repeat: _____ time(s).

Frequency: _____ x/day.

SPECIAL PROTOCOLS/NOTES: _____

_____

_____

PATIENT NAME: _____DATE:_____

THERAPIST NAME:_____

Unilateral Knee Flexion/Extension

PURPOSE: To increase range of motion and strengthen knee muscles.

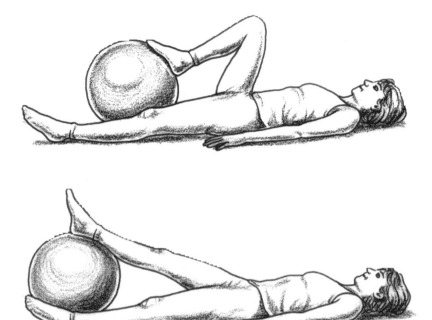

INSTRUCTION: Bend knee and place heel on ball. Straighten knee. Repeat with opposite side.

Hold: _____ second(s).   Repeat: _____ time(s).

Frequency: _____ x/day.

SPECIAL PROTOCOLS/NOTES: _____

_____

_____

PATIENT NAME: _____ DATE:_____

THERAPIST NAME:_____

Bilateral Knee Flexion/Extension

PURPOSE: To increase range of motion in hips.

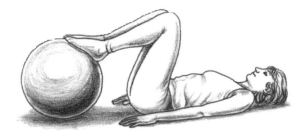

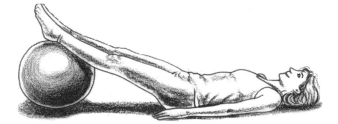

INSTRUCTION: Lie on back and place heels on ball. Bend both knees and draw up toward chest. Straighten knees.

Hold: _____ second(s).   Repeat: _____ time(s).

Frequency: _____ x/day.

SPECIAL PROTOCOLS/NOTES: _____

_____

_____

PATIENT NAME: _____DATE:_____

THERAPIST NAME:_____

Unilateral Knee Flexion/Extension with Ball against Wall

PURPOSE: To increase range of motion and strengthen knee and hip muscles.

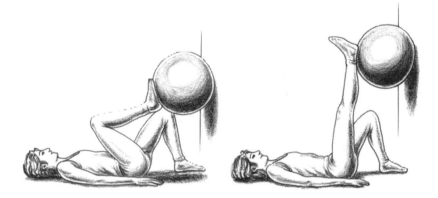

INSTRUCTION: Lie on back. Bend both knees. Place one foot on ball against wall. Extend leg. Repeat with opposite leg.

Hold: _____ second(s).   Repeat: _____ time(s).

Frequency: _____ x/day.

SPECIAL PROTOCOLS/NOTES: _____

_____

_____

PATIENT NAME: _____ DATE:_____

THERAPIST NAME:_____

Bilateral Knee Flexion/Extension with Ball against Wall

PURPOSE: To increase range of motion and strengthen knee and hip muscles.

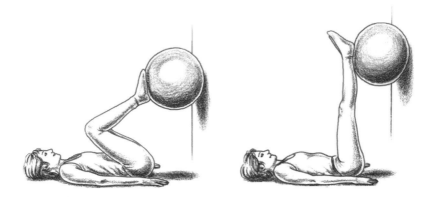

INSTRUCTION: Lie on back. Bend both knees. Place both feet on ball against wall. Extend both legs.

Hold: _____ second(s).   Repeat: _____ time(s).

Frequency: _____ x/day.

SPECIAL PROTOCOLS/NOTES: _____

_____

_____

PATIENT NAME: _____DATE:_____

THERAPIST NAME:_____

Bicycle

PURPOSE: To increase range of motion and strengthen hip and leg muscles.

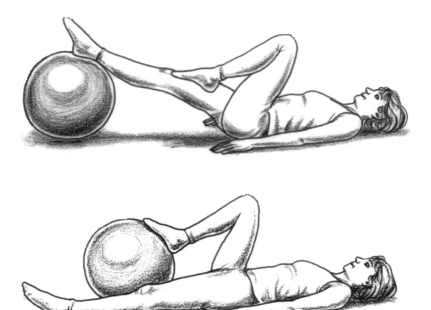

INSTRUCTION: Lie on back wth right leg straight and heel on ball. Bend left knee to chest. Then bend right knee, straighten left leg, and lower left leg to floor. Repeat with opposite side.

Repeat: _____ time(s).   Frequency: _____ x/day.

SPECIAL PROTOCOLS/NOTES: _____

_____

_____

PATIENT NAME: _____DATE:_____

THERAPIST NAME:_____

Bicycle

PURPOSE: To increase range of motion and strengthen abdominal, hip, and leg muscles. To improve coordination.

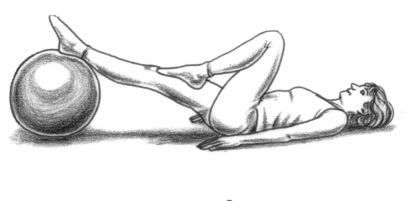

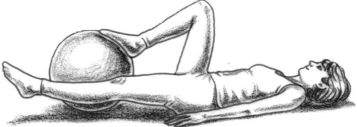

INSTRUCTION: Lie on back with right leg straight and heel on ball. Bend left knee to chest. Then bend right knee and straighten left leg. Do not let left leg touch floor. Repeat with opposite side.

Repeat: _____ time(s).   Frequency: _____ x/day.

SPECIAL PROTOCOLS/NOTES: __Do not arch back._____

_____

_____

PATIENT NAME: _____DATE:_____

THERAPIST NAME:_____

Bicycle

PURPOSE: To increase range of motion and strengthen abdominal, hip, and leg muscles. To improve coordination.

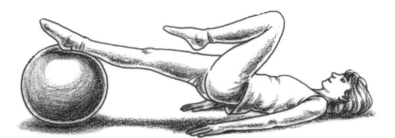

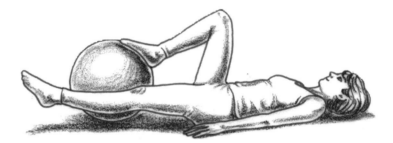

INSTRUCTION: Lie on back with right leg straight and heel on ball. Bend left knee to chest. Lift hips off floor. Then lower hips to floor, bend right knee to chest, and straighten left leg. Do not let left leg touch floor. Repeat with opposite side.

Repeat: _____ time(s).   Frequency: _____ x/day.

SPECIAL PROTOCOLS/NOTES: _____

_____

_____

PATIENT NAME: _____ DATE: _____

THERAPIST NAME: _____

Hip Abduction/Adduction with Hip Extension

PURPOSE: To strengthen buttock, hip, and inner and outer thigh muscles. To improve balance reactions.

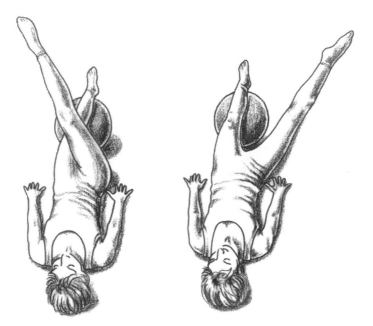

INSTRUCTION: Lie on back. Place ball under left leg. Extend both legs and lift hips off floor. Cross right leg over left leg. Uncross right leg and move away from body. Repeat with opposite side.

Repeat: _____ time(s).   Frequency: _____ x/day.

SPECIAL PROTOCOLS/NOTES: _Keep legs straight._____

_____

_____

PATIENT NAME: _____DATE:_____

THERAPIST NAME:_____

Hip Abduction/Adduction/
Extension to Figure "4"

PURPOSE: To strengthen buttock, hip, and leg muscles. To improve balance and coordination.

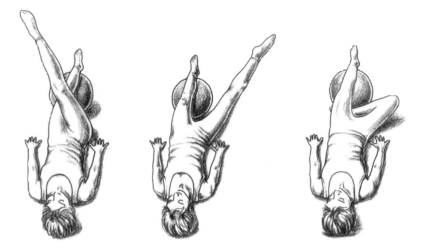

INSTRUCTION: Lie on back. Place ball under left leg. Extend both legs and hips off floor. Cross right leg over left leg. Uncross right leg, and move away from body. Then bend right knee and place right foot under left thigh. Repeat with opposite side.

Repeat: _____ time(s).   Frequency: _____ x/day.

SPECIAL PROTOCOLS/NOTES: Keep legs straight. _____

_____

_____

PATIENT NAME: _____ DATE:_____

THERAPIST NAME:_____

Unilateral Hip Abduction in Hooklying

PURPOSE: To strengthen abdominal and outer thigh muscles.

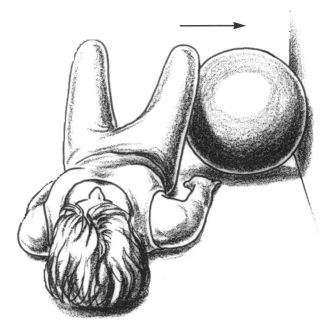

INSTRUCTION: Lie on back with body parallel to wall. Bend both knees. Place ball between knee and wall. Push knee against ball. Repeat with opposite side.

Hold: _____ second(s).   Repeat: _____ time(s).

Frequency: _____ x/day.

SPECIAL PROTOCOLS/NOTES: _____

_____

_____

PATIENT NAME: _____DATE:_____

THERAPIST NAME:_____

Lower Trunk Rotation in Hooklying

PURPOSE: To strengthen oblique abdominal muscles.

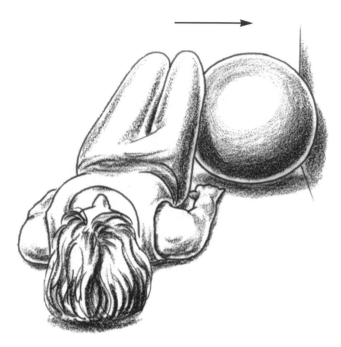

INSTRUCTION: Lie on back with body parallel to wall. Bend knees. Place ball between wall and knee. Push both knees against ball. Repeat with opposite side.

Hold: _____ second(s).   Repeat: _____ time(s).

Frequency: _____ x/day.

SPECIAL PROTOCOLS/NOTES: _____

_____

_____

PATIENT NAME: _____ DATE:_____

THERAPIST NAME:_____

Knee Adductor Squeeze in Hooklying

PURPOSE: To strengthen inner thigh muscles.

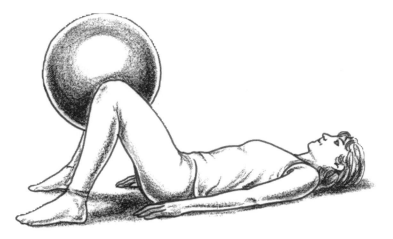

INSTRUCTION: Lie on back. Bend both knees with ball between knees. Squeeze ball.

Hold: _____ second(s).   Repeat: _____ time(s).

Frequency: _____ x/day.

SPECIAL PROTOCOLS/NOTES: _____

_____

_____

PATIENT NAME: _____ DATE:_____

THERAPIST NAME:_____

Knees to Chest
Ball between Knees

PURPOSE: To strengthen abdominal muscles.

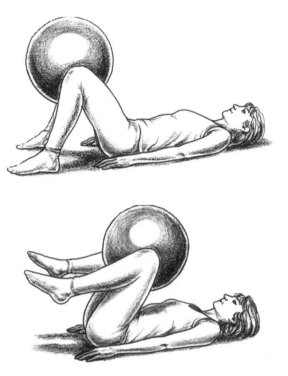

INSTRUCTION: Lie on back. Bend knees with ball between knees. Bring knees to chest.

Hold: _____ second(s).   Repeat: _____ time(s).

Frequency: _____ x/day.

SPECIAL PROTOCOLS/NOTES: _____

_____

_____

PATIENT NAME: _____DATE:_____

THERAPIST NAME:_____

Knees to Chest
Ball under Knees

PURPOSE: To strengthen abdominal muscles.

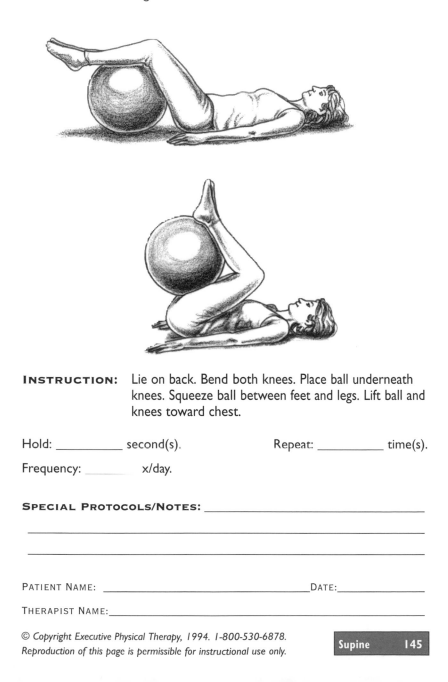

INSTRUCTION: Lie on back. Bend both knees. Place ball underneath knees. Squeeze ball between feet and legs. Lift ball and knees toward chest.

Hold: _____ second(s).   Repeat: _____ time(s).

Frequency: _____ x/day.

SPECIAL PROTOCOLS/NOTES: _____

_____

_____

PATIENT NAME: _____DATE:_____

THERAPIST NAME:_____

Knees to Chest
with Hands Overhead

PURPOSE: To strengthen abdominal and arm muscles.

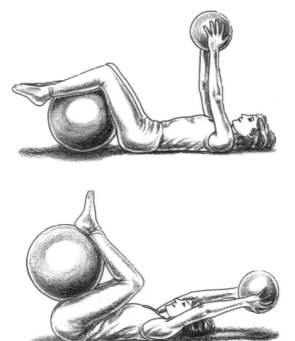

INSTRUCTION: Lie on back. Bend both knees. Place ball underneath knees. Place small ball between hands and extend arms up toward ceiling. Squeeze ball between feet and legs. Lift knees to chest and lower arms overhead.

Hold: _____ second(s).   Repeat: _____ time(s).

Frequency: _____ x/day.

SPECIAL PROTOCOLS/NOTES: _____

_____

_____

PATIENT NAME: _____ DATE:_____

THERAPIST NAME:_____

"Creager Crunch"

Purpose: To strengthen abdominal and arm muscles.

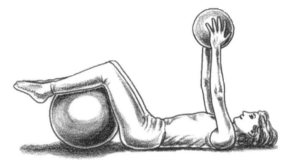

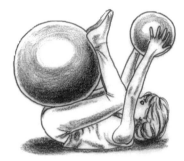

Instruction: Lie on back. Bend knees. Place ball underneath knees. Place small ball between hands. Extend arms overhead. Squeeze ball between feet and legs. Lift knees to chest and raise arms overhead.

Hold: _____ second(s).   Repeat: _____ time(s).

Frequency: _____ x/day.

Special Protocols/Notes: _____

_____

_____

Patient Name: _____Date:_____

Therapist Name:_____

Balance Ball on Feet

PURPOSE: To improve balance reactions and coordination.

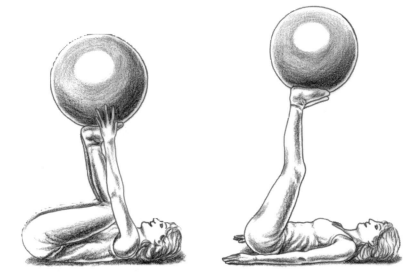

INSTRUCTION: Lie on back. Bend knees toward chest. Place ball on feet. Straighten knees and raise ball toward ceiling. Lower knees to chest.

Hold: _____ second(s).   Repeat: _____ time(s).

Frequency: _____ x/day.

SPECIAL PROTOCOLS/NOTES: _____

_____

_____

PATIENT NAME: _____DATE:_____

THERAPIST NAME:_____

Knee Flexion/Extension

PURPOSE: To stretch muscles in back of legs. To strengthen muscles in front of legs.

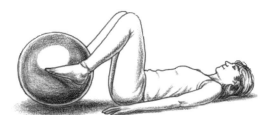

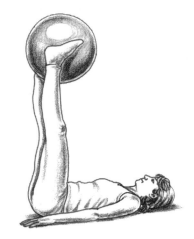

INSTRUCTION: Lie on back. Bend knees. Place ball between feet. Extend legs toward ceiling.

Hold: _____ second(s).   Repeat: _____ time(s).

Frequency: _____ x/day.

SPECIAL PROTOCOLS/NOTES: _Do not arch back when extending legs._

_____

_____

PATIENT NAME: _____ DATE:_____

THERAPIST NAME:_____

Internal/External Rotation of Legs

PURPOSE: To increase range of motion and strengthen inside and outside of leg and hip muscles. To strengthen abdominal muscles.

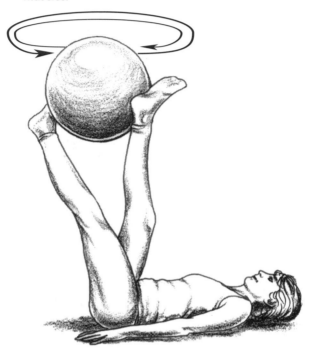

INSTRUCTION: Lie on back, bend knees, and lift legs toward ceiling. Rotate the ball between feet in both directions.

Repeat: _____ time(s).   Frequency: _____ x/day.

SPECIAL PROTOCOLS/NOTES: _____

_____

_____

PATIENT NAME: _____DATE:_____

THERAPIST NAME:_____

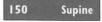

Supine with Legs Overhead

PURPOSE: To strengthen leg and abdominal muscles. To improve flexibility in the back and legs.

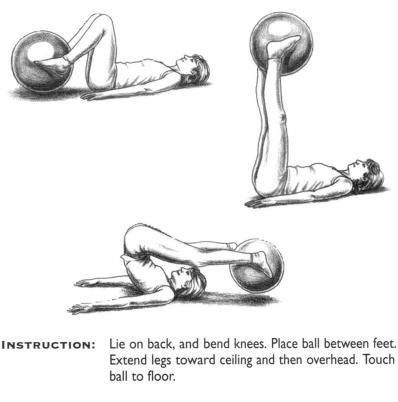

INSTRUCTION: Lie on back, and bend knees. Place ball between feet. Extend legs toward ceiling and then overhead. Touch ball to floor.

Hold: _____ second(s).   Repeat: _____ time(s).

Frequency: _____ x/day.

SPECIAL PROTOCOLS/NOTES: Keep arms on floor. _____

_____

_____

PATIENT NAME: _____ DATE: _____

THERAPIST NAME: _____

Trunk Extension
with Two Balls

PURPOSE: To strengthen abdominal, arm, back, leg, and neck muscles. To improve balance reactions.

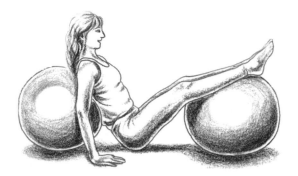

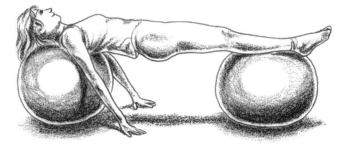

INSTRUCTION: Sit on floor. Place heels on one ball and lean against second ball. Lift hips off floor and rest head and shoulders on ball. Maintain body in straight line.

Hold: _____ second(s).   Repeat: _____ time(s).

Frequency: _____ x/day.

SPECIAL PROTOCOLS/NOTES: _____

_____

_____

PATIENT NAME: _____DATE:_____

THERAPIST NAME:_____

Trunk Extension and Hip Flexion with Two Balls

PURPOSE: To strengthen abdominal, arm, back, leg, and neck muscles. To improve balance reactions.

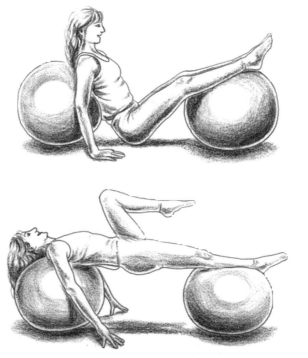

INSTRUCTION: Sit on floor. Place heels on one ball and lean against second ball. Lift hips off floor and rest head and shoulders on ball. Maintain body in straight line and bring one knee to chest. Repeat with opposite leg.

Hold: _____ second(s).   Repeat: _____ time(s).

Frequency: _____ x/day.

SPECIAL PROTOCOLS/NOTES: _____

_____

_____

PATIENT NAME: _____ DATE: _____

THERAPIST NAME: _____

Supine   153

CHAPTER FIVE

Bridge

Neutral in Bridge Position

PURPOSE: To strengthen muscles in an optimal position to prevent injury.

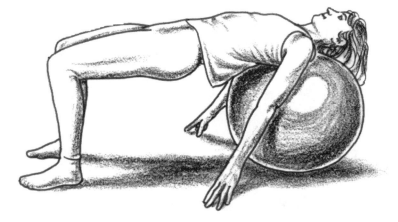

INSTRUCTION: Sit on ball. Walk legs out away from ball so head and shoulders rest on ball. Body is in bridged position. Rest hands on floor to help with balance.

Hold: _____ second(s).   Repeat: _____ time(s).

Frequency: _____ x/day.

SPECIAL PROTOCOLS/NOTES: _Do not arch back or let buttocks sag._

_____

_____

PATIENT NAME: _____DATE:_____

THERAPIST NAME:_____

Neutral in Bridge Position

PURPOSE: To strengthen muscles in an optimal position to prevent injury.

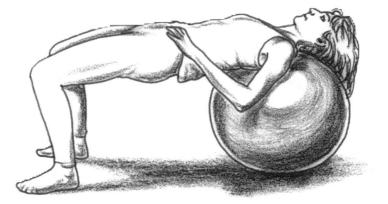

INSTRUCTION: Sit on ball. Walk legs out away from ball so head and shoulders rest on ball. Body is in bridge position.

Hold: _____ second(s).   Repeat: _____ time(s).

Frequency: _____ x/day.

SPECIAL PROTOCOLS/NOTES: Do not arch back or let buttocks sag.

_____

_____

PATIENT NAME: _____DATE:_____

THERAPIST NAME:_____

Heel Raises

PURPOSE: To strengthen calf, leg, back, and abdominal muscles. To improve balance reactions.

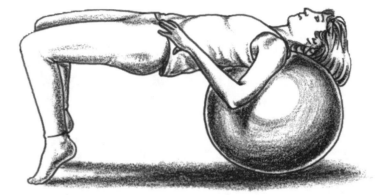

INSTRUCTION: Lie on ball in bridge position. Raise and lower heels. Keep toes on floor.

Hold: _____ second(s).   Repeat: _____ time(s).

Frequency: _____ x/day.

SPECIAL PROTOCOLS/NOTES: _____

_____

_____

PATIENT NAME: _____DATE:_____

THERAPIST NAME:_____

Hip Flexion

PURPOSE: To strengthen back, abdominal, and leg muscles. To improve balance reactions.

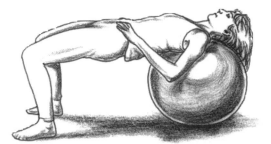

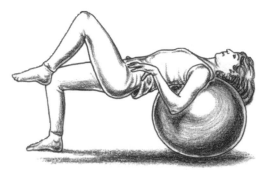

INSTRUCTION: Lie on ball in bridge position. Raise knee. Return to starting position. Repeat with opposite leg.

Hold: _____ second(s).   Repeat: _____ time(s).

Frequency: _____ x/day.

SPECIAL PROTOCOLS/NOTES: _____

_____

_____

PATIENT NAME: _____DATE:_____

THERAPIST NAME:_____

Knee Extension

PURPOSE: To strengthen back, leg, and abdominal muscles. To improve balance reactions.

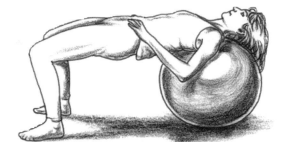

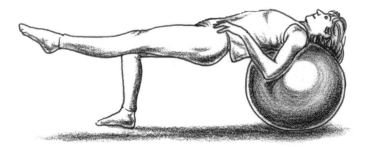

INSTRUCTION: Lie on ball in bridge position. Extend one leg. Return to starting position. Repeat with opposite leg.

Hold: _____ second(s).   Repeat: _____ time(s).

Frequency: _____ x/day.

SPECIAL PROTOCOLS/NOTES: _____

_____

_____

PATIENT NAME: _____ DATE: _____

THERAPIST NAME: _____

Write Alphabet with Foot

PURPOSE: To increase range of motion in foot. To strengthen foot, ankle, and leg muscles. To challenge balance reactions.

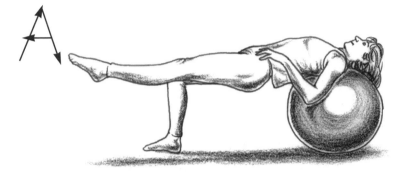

INSTRUCTION: Lie on ball in bridge position. Extend one leg. Write alphabet with foot. Repeat with opposite leg.

Repeat: _____ time(s).   Frequency: _____ x/day.

SPECIAL PROTOCOLS/NOTES: _____

_____

_____

PATIENT NAME: _____ DATE: _____

THERAPIST NAME: _____

Knee Flexion/Extension

PURPOSE: To strengthen hip, leg, back, and abdominal muscles. To improve balance reactions.

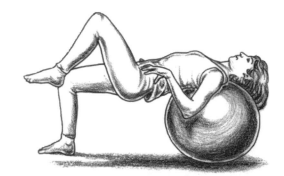

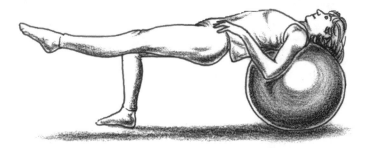

INSTRUCTION: Lie on ball in bridge position. Raise knee toward ceiling. Extend same leg. Repeat with opposite leg.

Hold: _____ second(s).   Repeat: _____ time(s).

Frequency: _____ x/day.

SPECIAL PROTOCOLS/NOTES: _____

_____

_____

PATIENT NAME: _____ DATE: _____

THERAPIST NAME: _____

Contralateral Shoulder and Hip Flexion

PURPOSE: To strengthen arm, leg, back, and abdominal muscles. To improve balance reactions.

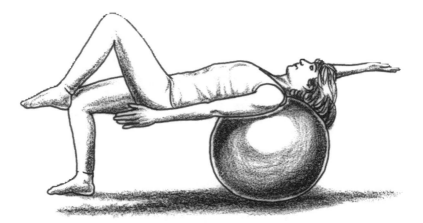

INSTRUCTION: Lie on ball in bridge position. Raise right arm overhead and left knee toward ceiling. Repeat with opposite side.

Hold: _____ second(s).   Repeat: _____ time(s).

Frequency: _____ x/day.

SPECIAL PROTOCOLS/NOTES: _____

_____

_____

PATIENT NAME: _____ DATE: _____

THERAPIST NAME: _____

Elbow Flexion/Extension

PURPOSE: To strengthen arm, leg, and back muscles. To improve balance reactions.

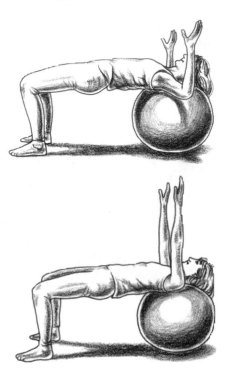

INSTRUCTION: Begin in bridge position. Bend elbows as shown. Raise arms toward ceiling.

Hold: _____ second(s).　　　　Repeat: _____ time(s).

Frequency: _____ x/day.

SPECIAL PROTOCOLS/NOTES: _____

_____

_____

PATIENT NAME: _____ DATE:_____

THERAPIST NAME:_____

Unilateral Shoulder Flexion

PURPOSE: To strengthen back, leg, shoulder, and abdominal muscles. To improve balance reactions.

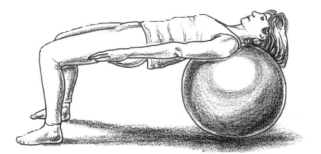

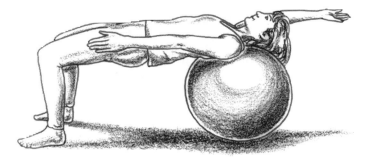

INSTRUCTION: Lie on ball in bridge position. Raise arm overhead. Repeat with opposite arm.

Hold: _____ second(s).   Repeat: _____ time(s).

Frequency: _____ x/day.

SPECIAL PROTOCOLS/NOTES: _____

_____

_____

PATIENT NAME: _____ DATE: _____

THERAPIST NAME: _____

Bilateral Shoulder Flexion

PURPOSE: To strengthen arm, back, leg, and abdominal muscles. To improve balance reactions.

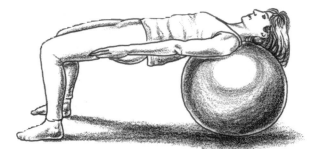

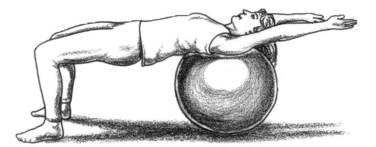

INSTRUCTION: Lie on ball in bridge position with arms by side of body. Raise both arms overhead.

Hold: _____ second(s).   Repeat: _____ time(s).

Frequency: _____ x/day.

SPECIAL PROTOCOLS/NOTES: _____

_____

_____

PATIENT NAME: _____ DATE:_____

THERAPIST NAME:_____

Bilateral Shoulder Flexion with Unilateral Hip Flexion

PURPOSE: To strengthen arm, hip, leg, back, and abdominal muscles. To improve balance reactions.

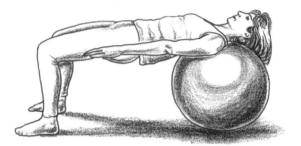

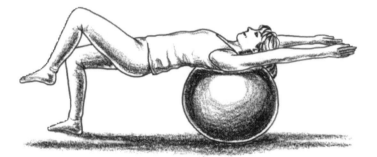

INSTRUCTION: Lie on ball in bridge position with arms by side of body. Raise arms overhead and one knee toward ceiling. Repeat with opposite knee.

Hold: _____ second(s).   Repeat: _____ time(s).

Frequency: _____ x/day.

SPECIAL PROTOCOLS/NOTES: _____

_____

_____

PATIENT NAME: _____ DATE:_____

THERAPIST NAME:_____

Bilateral Shoulder Flexion with Small Ball between Knees

PURPOSE: To strengthen arm, back, inner thigh, and abdominal muscles. To improve balance reactions.

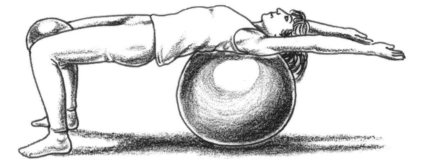

INSTRUCTION: Lie on ball in bridge position. Place ball between knees and squeeze lightly. Raise arms overhead.

Hold: _____ second(s).   Repeat: _____ time(s).

Frequency: _____ x/day.

SPECIAL PROTOCOLS/NOTES: _____

_____

_____

PATIENT NAME: _____ DATE: _____

THERAPIST NAME: _____

Cervical Flexion

PURPOSE: To strengthen neck muscles.

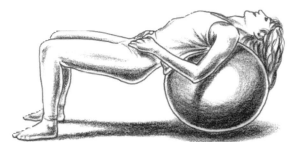

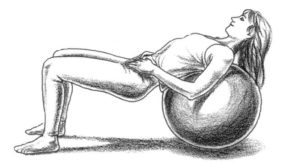

INSTRUCTION: Begin in bridge position. Let buttocks sag slightly. Raise head off ball.

Hold: _____ second(s).   Repeat: _____ time(s).

Frequency: _____ x/day.

SPECIAL PROTOCOLS/NOTES: _____

_____

_____

PATIENT NAME: _____ DATE:_____

THERAPIST NAME:_____

Horizontal Shoulder Adduction with Cervical Flexion

PURPOSE: To strengthen arm, leg, and neck muscles.

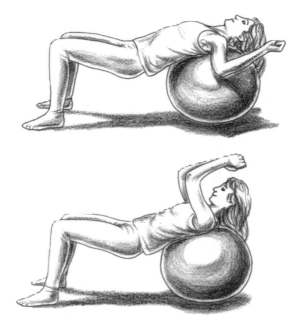

INSTRUCTION: Lie on ball in bridge position. Let hips sag. Bend elbows and lower arms to side of ball. Raise head off ball and touch forearms together. Lower head and arms.

Hold: _____ second(s).   Repeat: _____ time(s).

Frequency: _____ x/day.

SPECIAL PROTOCOLS/NOTES: _____

_____

_____

PATIENT NAME: _____DATE:_____

THERAPIST NAME:_____

Reclined Sit-Up

PURPOSE: To strengthen abdominal muscles.

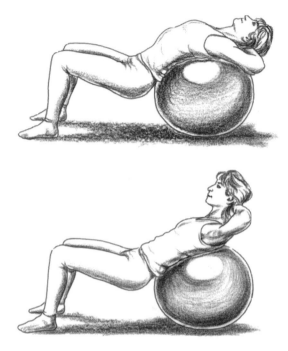

INSTRUCTION: Lie on ball in bridge position. Let hips sag. Place unclasped hands behind head. Lift head and elbows off ball.

Hold: _____ second(s).   Repeat: _____ time(s).

Frequency: _____ x/day.

SPECIAL PROTOCOLS/NOTES: _____

_____

_____

PATIENT NAME: _____DATE:_____

THERAPIST NAME:_____

Reclined Knee and Hip Flexion

PURPOSE: To strengthen abdominal and leg muscles. To improve balance reactions.

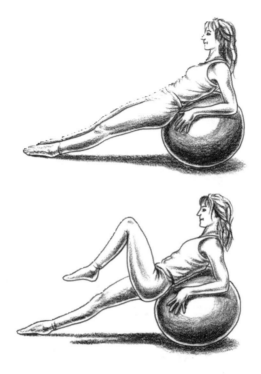

INSTRUCTION: Recline back on ball. Extend legs. Bend knee toward chest. Repeat with opposite knee.

Hold: _____ second(s).   Repeat: _____ time(s).

Frequency: _____ x/day.

SPECIAL PROTOCOLS/NOTES: _____

_____

_____

PATIENT NAME: _____DATE:_____

THERAPIST NAME:_____

Trunk Flexion/Extension with Feet on Ball

PURPOSE: To increase strength and range of motion in arm and shoulder muscles.

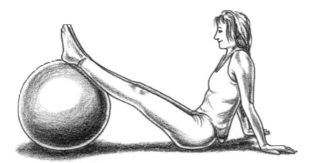

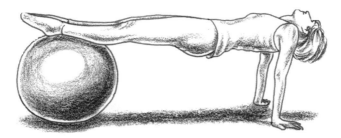

INSTRUCTION: Sit on floor. Place heels on ball. Straighten legs. Straighten arms and rotate hands so fingers point away from ball. Lift hips off floor. Keep body in straight line.

Hold: _____ second(s).   Repeat: _____ time(s).

Frequency: _____ x/day.

SPECIAL PROTOCOLS/NOTES: _____

_____

_____

PATIENT NAME: _____ DATE:_____

THERAPIST NAME:_____

Seated Squat to Bridge Position

PURPOSE: To stretch and strengthen hip and leg muscles.

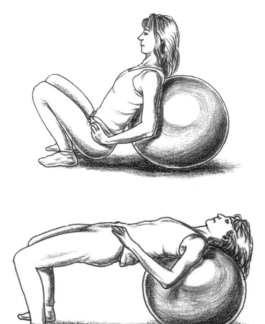

INSTRUCTION: Sit on floor. Place ball behind back. Lean against ball. Lift hips and rest head and shoulders on ball. Body is in bridge position.

Hold: _____ second(s).   Repeat: _____ time(s).

Frequency: _____ x/day.

SPECIAL PROTOCOLS/NOTES: _____

_____

_____

PATIENT NAME: _____DATE:_____

THERAPIST NAME:_____

Seated Squat against Ball

PURPOSE: To strengthen neck muscles. To improve posture.

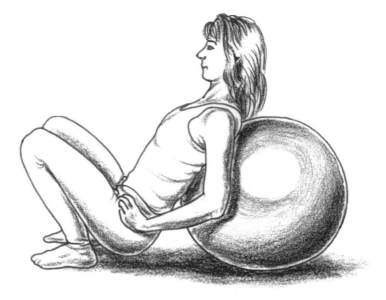

INSTRUCTION: Sit on floor. Place ball behind back. Lean against ball.
Keep head and shoulders in alignment.

Hold: _____ second(s).   Repeat: _____ time(s).

Frequency: _____ x/day.

SPECIAL PROTOCOLS/NOTES: Do not extend neck backward.

_____

_____

PATIENT NAME: _____DATE:_____

THERAPIST NAME:_____

Supine Leg Press

PURPOSE: To strengthen knee and leg muscles.

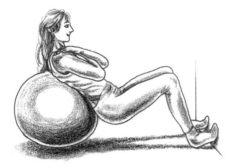

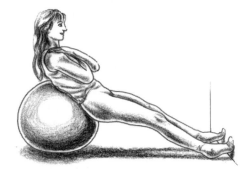

INSTRUCTION: Lean back against ball. Bend knees and place toes up against wall. Straighten legs as ball rolls backward.

Hold: _____ second(s).   Repeat: _____ time(s).

Frequency: _____ x/day.

SPECIAL PROTOCOLS/NOTES: _____

_____

_____

PATIENT NAME: _____ DATE: _____

THERAPIST NAME: _____

Quadriped

Neutral Position in Quadriped

PURPOSE: To strengthen muscles in an optimal position to avoid injury.

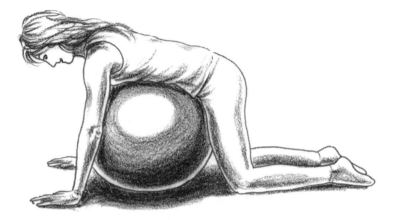

INSTRUCTION: Kneel. Lie with abdomen on ball. Maintain head alignment with body and natural curve in back.

Hold: _____ second(s).   Repeat: _____ time(s).

Frequency: _____ x/day.

SPECIAL PROTOCOLS/NOTES: Do not arch back or round back. _____

_____

_____

PATIENT NAME: _____DATE:_____

THERAPIST NAME:_____

Lateral Trunk Shifts

PURPOSE: To strengthen trunk muscles. To improve balance reactions.

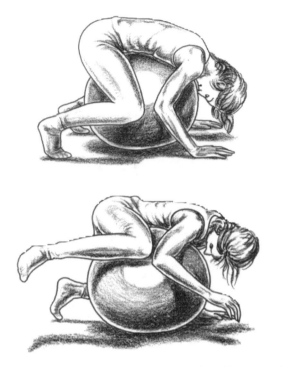

INSTRUCTION: Lie with abdomen on ball. Bend knees and place on each side of ball. Bend elbows and relax head down. Lift right hand and foot off floor and shift weight to left side. Repeat with opposite side.

Hold: _____ second(s).   Repeat: _____ time(s).

Frequency: _____ x/day.

SPECIAL PROTOCOLS/NOTES: _____

_____

_____

PATIENT NAME: _____ DATE:_____

THERAPIST NAME:_____

Shoulder Rowing

PURPOSE: To strengthen neck and mid-back shoulder muscles.

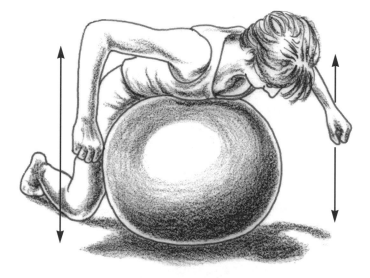

INSTRUCTION: Kneel. Lie with abdomen on ball. Bend elbows. Pull
elbows upward as if rowing.

Hold: _____ second(s).   Repeat: _____ time(s).

Frequency: _____ x/day.

SPECIAL PROTOCOLS/NOTES: _____

_____

_____

PATIENT NAME: _____DATE:_____

THERAPIST NAME:_____

Unilateral Shoulder Flexion

PURPOSE: To strengthen arm, neck, and shoulder muscles.

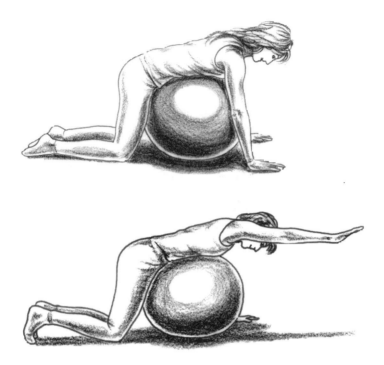

INSTRUCTION: Kneel. Lie with abdomen on ball. Raise one arm overhead. Repeat with opposite arm.

Hold: _____ second(s).   Repeat: _____ time(s).

Frequency: _____ x/day.

SPECIAL PROTOCOLS/NOTES: _____

_____

_____

PATIENT NAME: _____ DATE: _____

THERAPIST NAME: _____

Shoulder Flexion/Extension

PURPOSE: To increase range of motion and to strengthen shoulder and neck muscles.

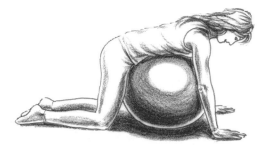

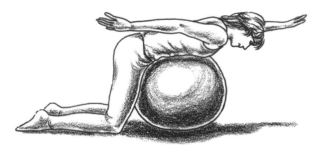

INSTRUCTION: Kneel. Lie with abdomen on ball. Raise one arm overhead and extend the other behind body. Alternate sides.

Hold: _____ second(s).   Repeat: _____ time(s).

Frequency: _____ x/day.

SPECIAL PROTOCOLS/NOTES: _____

_____

_____

PATIENT NAME: _____ DATE: _____

THERAPIST NAME: _____

Bilateral Shoulder Flexion

PURPOSE: To increase range of motion and strengthen arm and shoulder muscles. To strengthen neck muscles.

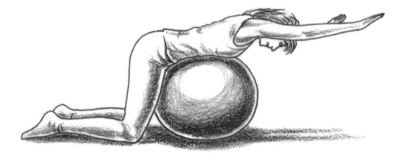

INSTRUCTION: Lie with abdomen on ball. Raise both arms overhead.

Hold: _____ second(s).   Repeat: _____ time(s).

Frequency: _____ x/day.

SPECIAL PROTOCOLS/NOTES: _____

_____

_____

PATIENT NAME: _____DATE:_____

THERAPIST NAME:_____

Unilateral Leg Extension

PURPOSE: To strengthen back, buttock, and leg muscles.

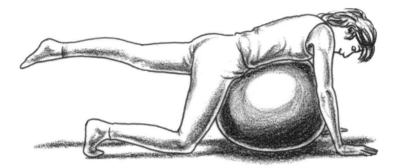

INSTRUCTION: Kneel. Lie with abdomen on ball. Extend one leg back. Repeat with opposite leg.

Hold: _____ second(s). Repeat: _____ time(s).

Frequency: _____ x/day.

SPECIAL PROTOCOLS/NOTES: _____

_____

_____

PATIENT NAME: _____DATE:_____

THERAPIST NAME:_____

Contralateral Shoulder Flexion and Leg Extension

PURPOSE: To strengthen arm, back, neck, and leg muscles.

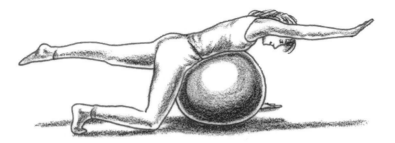

INSTRUCTION: Kneel. Lie with abdomen on ball. Extend one leg back and opposite arm overhead. Repeat with opposite arm and leg.

Hold: _____ second(s). Repeat: _____ time(s).

Frequency: _____ x/day.

SPECIAL PROTOCOLS/NOTES: _____

_____

_____

PATIENT NAME: _____ DATE:_____

THERAPIST NAME:_____

Trunk Rotation

PURPOSE: To strengthen arm muscles. To improve trunk flexibility.

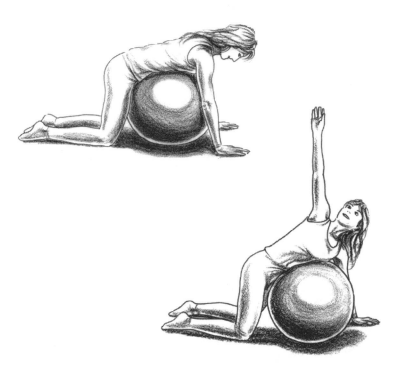

INSTRUCTION: Kneel. Lie with abdomen on ball. Lift one arm out to side of body. Rotate torso as arm is raised to ceiling. Watch hand throughout motion. Repeat with opposite side.

Hold: _____ second(s).   Repeat: _____ time(s).

Frequency: _____ x/day.

SPECIAL PROTOCOLS/NOTES: _____

_____

_____

PATIENT NAME: _____ DATE: _____

THERAPIST NAME: _____

Trunk Extension

PURPOSE: To strengthen arm, back, and neck muscles.

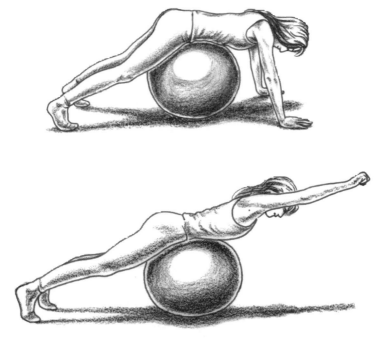

INSTRUCTION: Lie with abdomen on ball. Raise trunk and arms up. Keep head aligned between arms.

Hold: _____ second(s).   Repeat: _____ time(s).

Frequency: _____ x/day.

SPECIAL PROTOCOLS/NOTES: _____

_____

_____

PATIENT NAME: _____DATE:_____

THERAPIST NAME:_____

Trunk Extension

PURPOSE: To strengthen neck and back muscles.

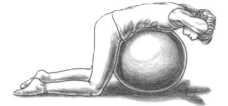

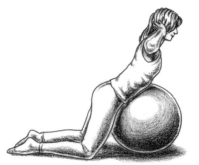

INSTRUCTION: Lie with abdomen on ball and knees on floor. Place unclasped hands behind head. Lift head, shoulders, and chest off ball.

Hold: _____ second(s).   Repeat: _____ time(s).

Frequency: _____ x/day.

SPECIAL PROTOCOLS/NOTES: _____

_____

_____

PATIENT NAME: _____ DATE: _____

THERAPIST NAME: _____

Cervical Flexion

PURPOSE: To strengthen neck muscles.

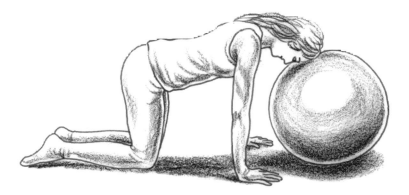

INSTRUCTION: Begin with hands and knees on floor. Place ball underneath forehead. Lightly press forehead into ball.

Hold: _____ second(s).   Repeat: _____ time(s).

Frequency: _____ x/day.

SPECIAL PROTOCOLS/NOTES: _____

_____

_____

PATIENT NAME: _____ DATE: _____

THERAPIST NAME: _____

Cervical and Unilateral Shoulder Flexion

PURPOSE: To strengthen arm and neck muscles.

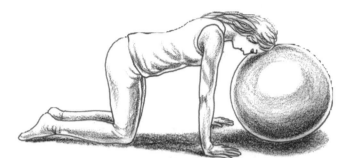

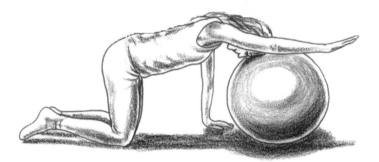

INSTRUCTION: Begin with hands and knees on floor. Place ball underneath forehead. Raise one arm. Repeat with opposite arm.

Hold: _____ second(s).   Repeat: _____ time(s).

Frequency: _____ x/day.

SPECIAL PROTOCOLS/NOTES: _____

_____

_____

PATIENT NAME: _____ DATE:_____

THERAPIST NAME:_____

Cervical and Bilateral Shoulder Flexion

PURPOSE: To strengthen arm and neck muscles.

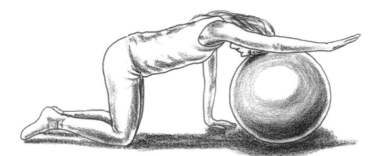

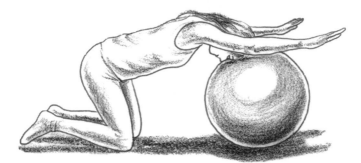

INSTRUCTION: Begin with hands and feet on floor. Place ball underneath forehead. Raise both arms.

Hold: _____ second(s).   Repeat: _____ time(s).

Frequency: _____ x/day.

SPECIAL PROTOCOLS/NOTES: _____

_____

_____

PATIENT NAME: _____ DATE:_____

THERAPIST NAME:_____

Unilateral Knee Flexion and Hip Extension

PURPOSE: To strengthen arm, back, buttock, and leg muscles.

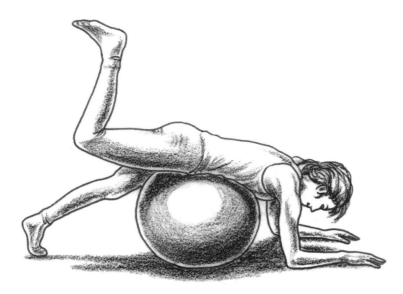

INSTRUCTION: Lie with abdomen on ball. Lean forward and place forearms on floor. Bend one knee and lift foot toward ceiling. Repeat with opposite leg.

Hold: _____ second(s).   Repeat: _____ time(s).

Frequency: _____ x/day.

SPECIAL PROTOCOLS/NOTES: __Do not arch back._____

_____

_____

PATIENT NAME: _____DATE:_____

THERAPIST NAME:_____

Bilateral Knee Flexion and Hip Extension

PURPOSE: To strengthen arm, back, buttock, and leg muscles.

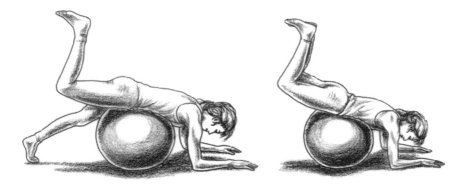

INSTRUCTION: Lie with abdomen on ball. Lean forward and place forearms on floor. Bend one knee and lift foot toward ceiling. Bend opposite knee and lift foot toward ceiling.

Hold: _____ second(s).   Repeat: _____ time(s).

Frequency: _____ x/day.

SPECIAL PROTOCOLS/NOTES: _____

_____

_____

PATIENT NAME: _____ DATE:_____

THERAPIST NAME:_____

Hip Extension
with Knee Flexion

PURPOSE: To strengthen arm, buttock, and leg muscles. To increase range of motion in hips.

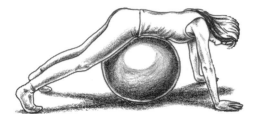

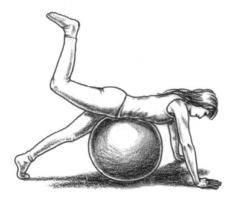

INSTRUCTION: Lie with ball under abdomen. Bend one knee and lift foot toward ceiling. Repeat with opposite leg.

Hold: _____ second(s).   Repeat: _____ time(s).

Frequency: _____ x/day.

SPECIAL PROTOCOLS/NOTES: ___Do not arch back when lifting foot___
___toward ceiling._____

_____

PATIENT NAME: _____DATE:_____

THERAPIST NAME:_____

Lumbar Lordosis

PURPOSE: To increase low back range of motion.

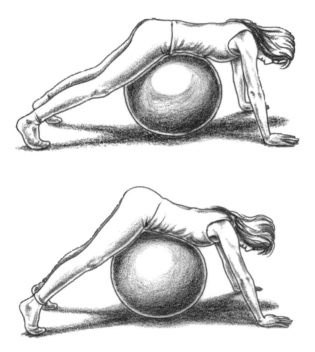

INSTRUCTION: Place ball under abdomen. Lift buttocks toward ceiling.

Hold: _____ second(s).   Repeat: _____ time(s).

Frequency: _____ x/day.

SPECIAL PROTOCOLS/NOTES: _____

_____

_____

PATIENT NAME: _____ DATE:_____

THERAPIST NAME:_____

© *Copyright Executive Physical Therapy, 1994. 1-800-530-6878.*
Reproduction of this page is permissible for instructional use only.

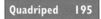

Quadriped   195

Praying Mantis

PURPOSE: To strengthen abdominal, back, and shoulder muscles.

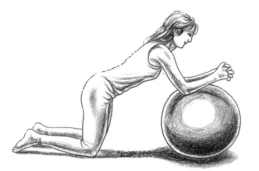

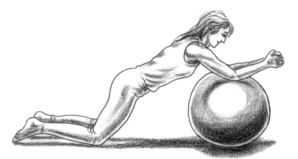

INSTRUCTION: Kneel. Clasp hands. Lean forward and place bent elbows on ball. Roll ball forward with elbows. Return to starting position.

Hold: _____ second(s).   Repeat: _____ time(s).

Frequency: _____ x/day.

SPECIAL PROTOCOLS/NOTES: _____

_____

_____

PATIENT NAME: _____ DATE:_____

THERAPIST NAME:_____

CHAPTER SEVEN
Prone

Neutral Position in Prone

PURPOSE: To strengthen muscles in an optimal position to prevent injury.

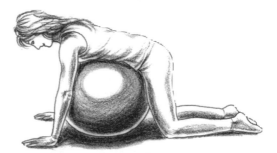

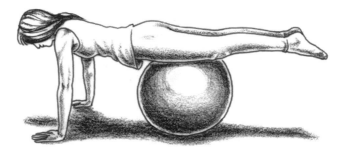

INSTRUCTION: Kneel. Lie with abdomen on ball. Walk arms out until thighs are on ball.

Hold: _____ second(s).   Repeat: _____ time(s).

Frequency: _____ x/day.

SPECIAL PROTOCOLS/NOTES: Do not let abdomen sag. _____

_____

_____

PATIENT NAME: _____ DATE:_____

THERAPIST NAME:_____

Prone Walk-Out

PURPOSE: To strengthen arm and shoulder muscles. To improve balance reactions.

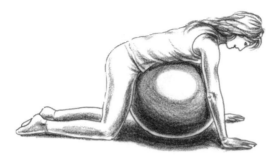

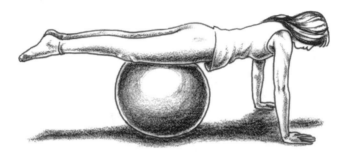

INSTRUCTION: Begin in neutral position. Walk arms out until ball is under thighs.

Hold: _____ second(s).   Repeat: _____ time(s).

Frequency: _____ x/day.

SPECIAL PROTOCOLS/NOTES: Do not let abdomen sag. _____

_____

_____

PATIENT NAME: _____ DATE: _____

THERAPIST NAME: _____

ADVANCED
Prone Walk-Out

PURPOSE: To strengthen arm and shoulder muscles. To improve balance reactions.

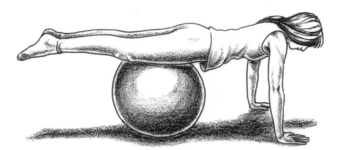

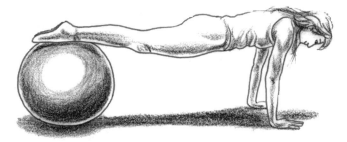

INSTRUCTION: Begin in neutral position. Walk arms out until feet are on ball.

Hold: _____ second(s).   Repeat: _____ time(s).

Frequency: _____ x/day.

SPECIAL PROTOCOLS/NOTES: Do not let abdomen sag. _____

_____

_____

PATIENT NAME: _____ DATE: _____

THERAPIST NAME: _____

Legs Side to Side

PURPOSE: To strengthen abdominal, arm, shoulder, and leg muscles. To improve balance reactions.

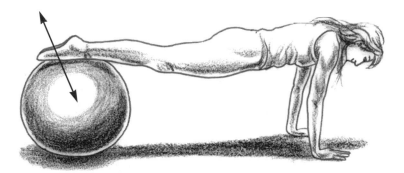

INSTRUCTION: Begin in neutral position. Walk arms out until feet are on ball. Roll ball slightly from side to side with feet.

Hold: _____ second(s).   Repeat: _____ time(s).

Frequency: _____ x/day.

SPECIAL PROTOCOLS/NOTES: _____

_____

_____

PATIENT NAME: _____ DATE:_____

THERAPIST NAME:_____

Hip Extension

PURPOSE: To strengthen abdominal, arm, back, buttock, and leg muscles. To improve balance reactions.

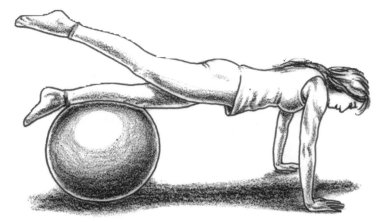

INSTRUCTION: Begin in neutral position. Walk arms out until feet are on ball. Keep legs straight and lift one up toward ceiling. Repeat with other leg.

Hold: _____ second(s).   Repeat: _____ time(s).

Frequency: _____ x/day.

SPECIAL PROTOCOLS/NOTES: __Do not lift leg so high that back arches.__

_____

_____

PATIENT NAME: _____DATE:_____

THERAPIST NAME:_____

Lower Body Extension

PURPOSE: To strengthen abdominal, arm, and leg muscles. To improve balance reactions.

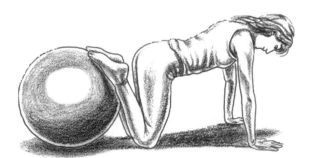

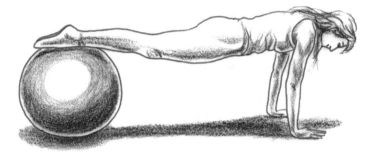

INSTRUCTION: Begin on hands and knees. Lift feet up and place on top of ball. Extend legs out to neutral position.

Hold: _____ second(s).   Repeat: _____ time(s).

Frequency: _____ x/day.

SPECIAL PROTOCOLS/NOTES: _____

_____

_____

PATIENT NAME: _____ DATE: _____

THERAPIST NAME: _____

Abdominal Dips

PURPOSE: To strengthen abdominal muscles.

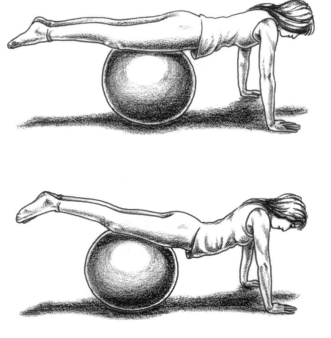

INSTRUCTION: Begin in neutral position with thighs on ball. Lower abdomen toward floor. Return to starting position.

Repeat: _____ time(s).   Frequency: _____ x/day.

SPECIAL PROTOCOLS/NOTES: __Do exercise slowly._____

_____

_____

PATIENT NAME: _____ DATE:_____

THERAPIST NAME:_____

Pelvic Clock

PURPOSE: To strengthen abdominal, arm, and back muscles. To challenge balance reactions.

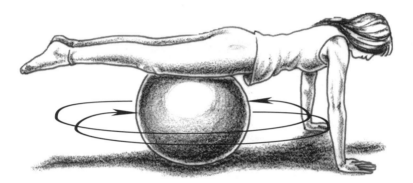

INSTRUCTION: Begin in neutral position. Make small circles with abdominal muscles, clockwise and counter-clockwise.

Hold: _____ second(s).   Repeat: _____ time(s).

Frequency: _____ x/day.

SPECIAL PROTOCOLS/NOTES: __Do not bend hips._____

_____

_____

PATIENT NAME: _____ DATE:_____

THERAPIST NAME:_____

Unilateral Shoulder Flexion

PURPOSE: To increase range of motion and strengthen arm and shoulder muscles.

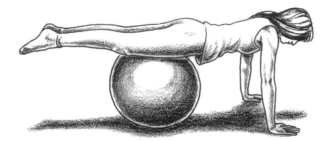

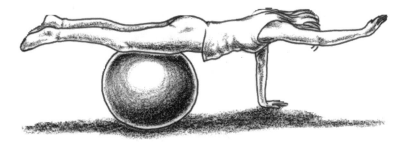

INSTRUCTION: Begin in neutral position. Walk arms out until thighs are on ball. Lift one arm up toward ceiling. Repeat with other arm.

Hold: _____ second(s).   Repeat: _____ time(s).

Frequency: _____ x/day.

SPECIAL PROTOCOLS/NOTES: _Do not arch back._ _____

_____

_____

PATIENT NAME: _____ DATE:_____

THERAPIST NAME:_____

Push-Up

PURPOSE: To strengthen arm muscles. To improve balance reactions.

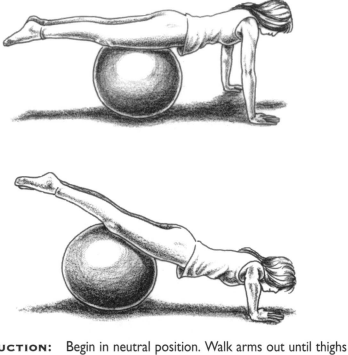

INSTRUCTION: Begin in neutral position. Walk arms out until thighs are on ball. Do a push-up.

Hold: _____ second(s).   Repeat: _____ time(s).

Frequency: _____ x/day.

SPECIAL PROTOCOLS/NOTES: __Do not let abdomen sag._____

_____

_____

PATIENT NAME: _____DATE:_____

THERAPIST NAME:_____

Push-Up on Ball

PURPOSE: To strengthen shoulder muscles. To improve balance reactions.

INSTRUCTION: Lie with abdomen on ball, legs extended, and toes on floor. Bend elbows and place one hand on each side of ball. Extend arms into push-up position.

Hold: _____ second(s).   Repeat: _____ time(s).

Frequency: _____ x/day.

SPECIAL PROTOCOLS/NOTES: _____

_____

_____

PATIENT NAME: _____DATE:_____

THERAPIST NAME:_____

Abdominal Crunch

PURPOSE: To strengthen arm and abdominal muscles.

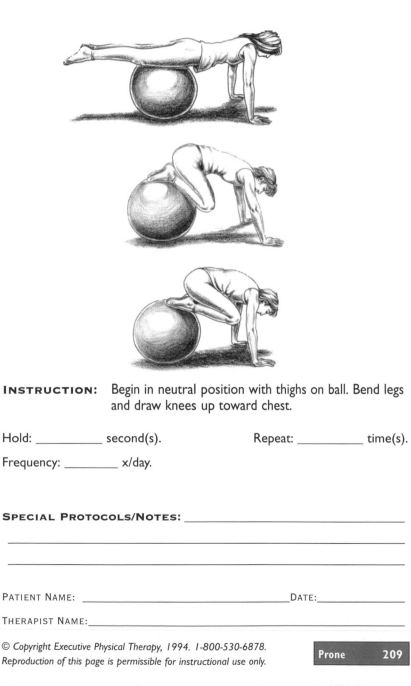

INSTRUCTION: Begin in neutral position with thighs on ball. Bend legs and draw knees up toward chest.

Hold: _____ second(s).   Repeat: _____ time(s).

Frequency: _____ x/day.

SPECIAL PROTOCOLS/NOTES: _____

_____

_____

PATIENT NAME: _____ DATE: _____

THERAPIST NAME: _____

Prone Tucks

PURPOSE: To increase back flexibility. To strengthen abdominal, arm, and neck muscles.

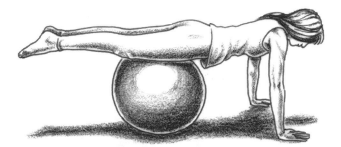

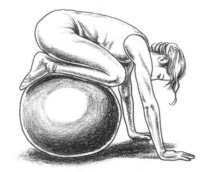

INSTRUCTION: Lie on ball in push-up position with ball under thighs. Bring knees to chest until body is in a tuck position.

Hold: _____ second(s).   Repeat: _____ time(s).

Frequency: _____ x/day.

SPECIAL PROTOCOLS/NOTES: _____

_____

_____

PATIENT NAME: _____DATE:_____

THERAPIST NAME:_____

The Skier

PURPOSE: To increase back and hip flexibility. To strengthen abdominal, arm, back, and neck muscles.

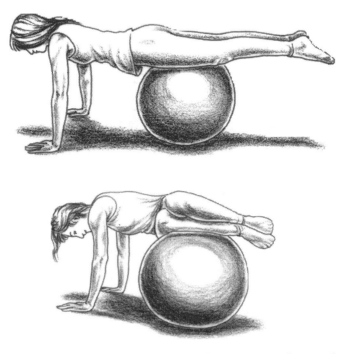

INSTRUCTION: Begin in neutral position. Bend knees and rotate hips so right outer ankle is touching ball. Draw legs up to chest on left side. Repeat with opposite side.

Hold: _____ second(s).   Repeat: _____ time(s).

Frequency: _____ x/day.

SPECIAL PROTOCOLS/NOTES: _____

_____

_____

PATIENT NAME: _____DATE:_____

THERAPIST NAME:_____

The Scissors

PURPOSE: To strengthen abdominal, arm, back, leg, and neck muscles. To improve coordination of upper and lower body. To challenge balance reactions.

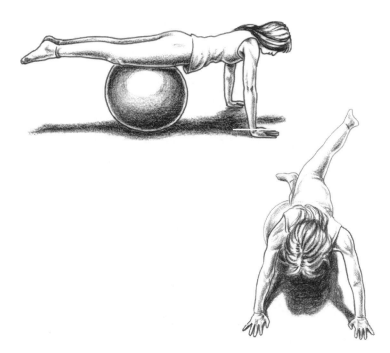

INSTRUCTION: Begin in neutral position with ball under thighs. Keep legs straight. Lift one leg up toward ceiling and rotate over opposite leg. Repeat with opposite side.

Hold: _____ second(s).   Repeat: _____ time(s).

Frequency: _____ x/day.

SPECIAL PROTOCOLS/NOTES: ___Eyes should be focused on floor.___
___Maintain head in alignment with shoulders._____

_____

PATIENT NAME: _____DATE:_____

THERAPIST NAME:_____

The Diver

PURPOSE: To strengthen arm, back, leg, and neck muscles. To improve balance reactions and coordination.

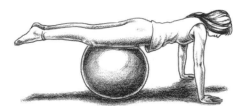

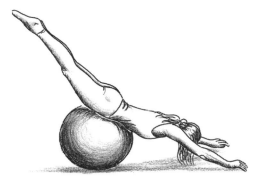

INSTRUCTION: Lie on ball in push-up position. Push ball back with hips and lift legs up toward ceiling.

Hold: _____ second(s).   Repeat: _____ time(s).

Frequency: _____ x/day.

SPECIAL PROTOCOLS/NOTES: _Keep arms straight throughout_ exercise. _____

_____

PATIENT NAME: _____ DATE:_____

THERAPIST NAME:_____

Tuck Position into the Diver Position

PURPOSE: To increase flexibility in back. To strengthen abdominal, arm, back, leg, and neck muscles. To improve balance reactions and coordination.

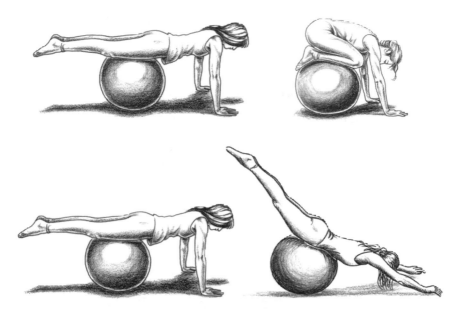

INSTRUCTION: Lie on ball in neutral position with ball under thighs. Bring knees to chest until body is in tuck position. Return to push-up position. Push ball back with hips and lift legs up toward ceiling.

Hold: _____ second(s).   Repeat: _____ time(s).

Frequency: _____ x/day.

SPECIAL PROTOCOLS/NOTES: _____

_____

_____

PATIENT NAME: _____ DATE: _____

THERAPIST NAME: _____

The Ferris Wheel

PURPOSE: To strengthen arm, back, leg, and neck muscles. To improve balance reactions and coordination.

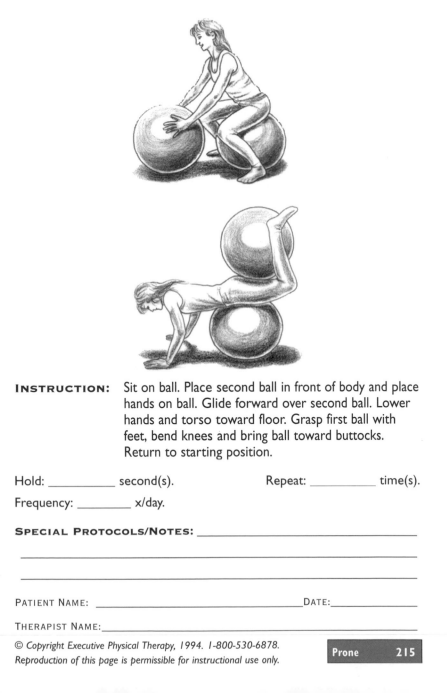

INSTRUCTION: Sit on ball. Place second ball in front of body and place hands on ball. Glide forward over second ball. Lower hands and torso toward floor. Grasp first ball with feet, bend knees and bring ball toward buttocks. Return to starting position.

Hold: _____ second(s).   Repeat: _____ time(s).

Frequency: _____ x/day.

SPECIAL PROTOCOLS/NOTES: _____

_____

_____

PATIENT NAME: _____ DATE:_____

THERAPIST NAME:_____

Neutral Position in Prone on Floor

PURPOSE: To strengthen muscles in an optimal position to avoid injury.

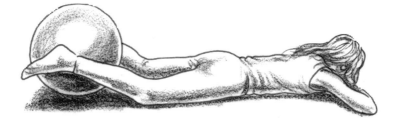

INSTRUCTION: Lie on abdomen. Hold ball between feet.

Hold: _____ second(s).   Repeat: _____ time(s).

Frequency: _____ x/day.

SPECIAL PROTOCOLS/NOTES: _____

_____

_____

PATIENT NAME: _____DATE:_____

THERAPIST NAME:_____

Prone Unilateral Knee and Hip Extension

PURPOSE: To increase range of motion and strengthen knee and hip muscles.

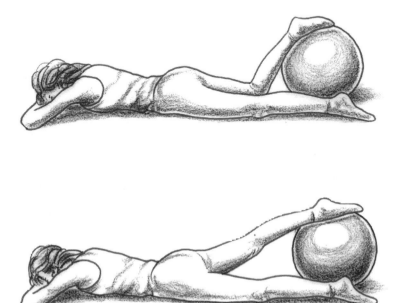

INSTRUCTION: Lie on abdomen. Place one foot on ball. Straighten leg. Repeat with opposite side.

Hold: _____ second(s).   Repeat: _____ time(s).

Frequency: _____ x/day.

SPECIAL PROTOCOLS/NOTES: _____

_____

_____

PATIENT NAME: _____DATE:_____

THERAPIST NAME:_____

Bilateral Knee and Hip Extension

PURPOSE: To increase range of motion and strengthen knee and hip muscles.

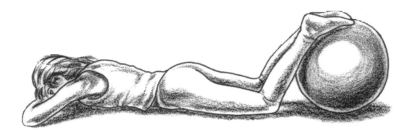

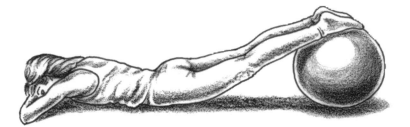

INSTRUCTION: Lie on abdomen. Place feet on ball. Straighten both legs.

Hold: _____ second(s).   Repeat: _____ time(s).

Frequency: _____ x/day.

SPECIAL PROTOCOLS/NOTES: _____

_____

_____

PATIENT NAME: _____DATE:_____

THERAPIST NAME:_____

Ankle Squeeze

PURPOSE: To strengthen inner leg and thigh muscles.

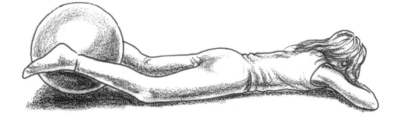

INSTRUCTION: Lie on abdomen. Place ball between feet. Squeeze
ankles together.

Hold: _____ second(s).   Repeat: _____ time(s).

Frequency: _____ x/day.

SPECIAL PROTOCOLS/NOTES: _____

_____

_____

PATIENT NAME: _____DATE:_____

THERAPIST NAME:_____

Knee Flexion

PURPOSE: To strengthen knee and leg muscles.

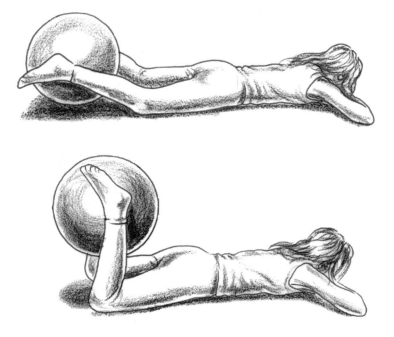

INSTRUCTION: Lie on abdomen. Place ball between feet. Bend knees and bring ball toward buttocks.

Hold: _____ second(s).   Repeat: _____ time(s).

Frequency: _____ x/day.

SPECIAL PROTOCOLS/NOTES: _____

_____

_____

PATIENT NAME: _____DATE:_____

THERAPIST NAME:_____

Trunk Extension

PURPOSE: To strengthen arm, back, and neck muscles.

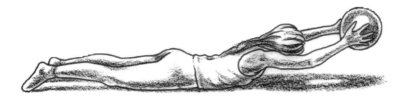

INSTRUCTION: Lie on abdomen. Place small ball between hands. Straighten arms overhead. Lift arms and chest off floor. Keep head between arms.

Hold: _____ second(s).   Repeat: _____ time(s).

Frequency: _____ x/day.

SPECIAL PROTOCOLS/NOTES: _____

_____

_____

PATIENT NAME: _____ DATE:_____

THERAPIST NAME:_____

CHAPTER EIGHT
Sidelying

Knee Flexion/Extension

PURPOSE: To increase range of motion and strengthen knee muscles.

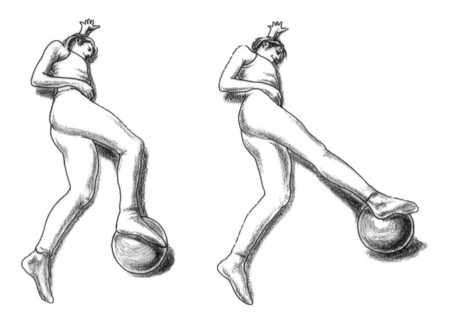

INSTRUCTION: Lie on side with bottom knee bent. Place top foot on ball. Extend knee. Repeat with opposite side.

Hold: _____ second(s).   Repeat: _____ time(s).

Frequency: _____ x/day.

SPECIAL PROTOCOLS/NOTES: _____

_____

_____

PATIENT NAME: _____ DATE: _____

THERAPIST NAME: _____

Hip Flexion

PURPOSE: To increase range of motion and strengthen hip muscles.

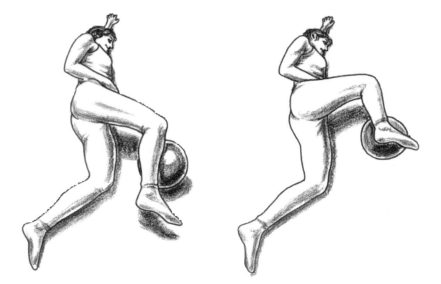

INSTRUCTION: Lie on side with bottom knee bent. Place top leg on ball. Flex knee toward chest. Repeat with opposite side.

Hold: _____ second(s).   Repeat: _____ time(s).

Frequency: _____ x/day.

SPECIAL PROTOCOLS/NOTES: _____

_____

_____

PATIENT NAME: _____ DATE:_____

THERAPIST NAME:_____

Hip Extension

PURPOSE: To increase range of motion and strengthen hip muscles.

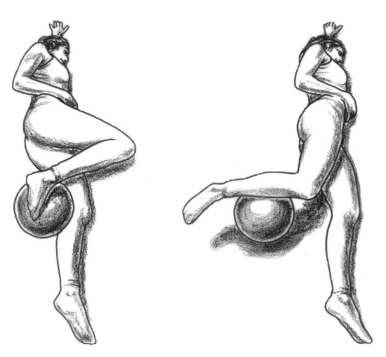

INSTRUCTION: Lie on side. Bend top knee and place foot on ball. Extend leg behind body. Repeat with opposite side.

Hold: _____ second(s).   Repeat: _____ time(s).

Frequency: _____ x/day.

SPECIAL PROTOCOLS/NOTES: _____

_____

_____

PATIENT NAME: _____DATE:_____

THERAPIST NAME:_____

Shoulder Flexion/Extension

PURPOSE: To increase range of motion and strengthen shoulder muscles.

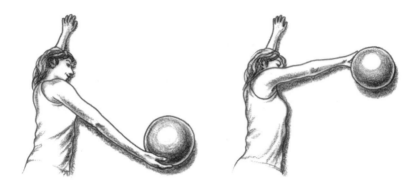

INSTRUCTION: Lie on side. Extend arm and place hand on ball. Roll ball toward head and down toward hip. Repeat with opposite side.

Repeat: _____ time(s).   Frequency: _____ x/day.

SPECIAL PROTOCOLS/NOTES: _____

_____

_____

PATIENT NAME: _____ DATE:_____

THERAPIST NAME:_____

Shoulder
Protraction/Retraction

PURPOSE: To increase range of motion and strengthen shoulder muscles.

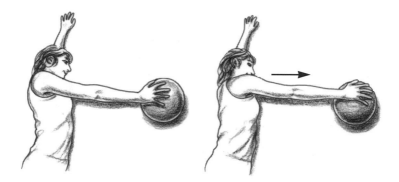

INSTRUCTION: Lie on side. Extend arm out away from body. Place ball under hand. Gently push ball out with shoulder. Repeat with opposite side.

Repeat: _____ time(s).   Frequency: _____ x/day.

SPECIAL PROTOCOLS/NOTES: ___Do not bend elbow during exercise.___

_____

_____

PATIENT NAME: _____ DATE:_____

THERAPIST NAME:_____

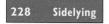

Hip Adductor Squeeze

PURPOSE: To strengthen inner thigh muscles.

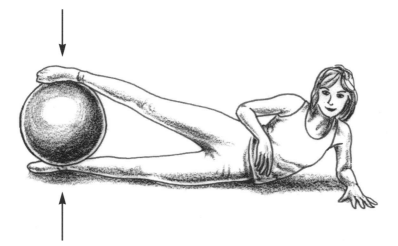

INSTRUCTION: Lie on side. Place ball between feet. Squeeze ball.
Repeat with opposite side.

Hold: _____ second(s).   Repeat: _____ time(s).

Frequency: _____ x/day.

SPECIAL PROTOCOLS/NOTES: _____

_____

_____

PATIENT NAME: _____DATE:_____

THERAPIST NAME:_____

Hip Adductor/Abductor Lift

PURPOSE: To strengthen inner and outer thigh muscles.

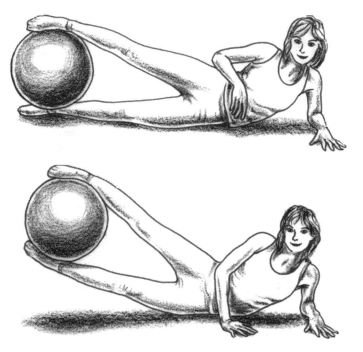

INSTRUCTION: Lie on side. Place ball between feet. Lift legs toward ceiling. Repeat with opposite side.

Hold: _____ second(s).   Repeat: _____ time(s).

Frequency: _____ x/day.

SPECIAL PROTOCOLS/NOTES: _____

_____

_____

PATIENT NAME: _____ DATE: _____

THERAPIST NAME: _____

1-800-530-6878. © Copyright Executive Physical Therapy, 1994.
Reproduction of this page is permissible for instructional use only.

Standing

Bounce Ball with Hand

PURPOSE: To improve coordination.

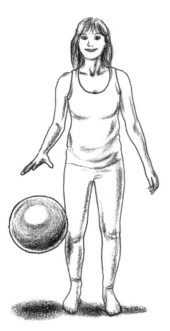

INSTRUCTION: Stand. Bounce ball with hand. Repeat with opposite hand.

Hold: _____ second(s).   Repeat: _____ time(s).

Frequency: _____ x/day.

SPECIAL PROTOCOLS/NOTES: Keep eyes looking forward. _____

_____

_____

PATIENT NAME: _____DATE:_____

THERAPIST NAME:_____

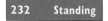

Walk and Bounce Ball
with Hand

PURPOSE: To improve coordination.

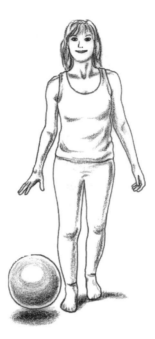

INSTRUCTION: Walk and bounce ball with hand. Repeat with opposite
hand.

Hold: _____ second(s).   Repeat: _____ time(s).

Frequency: _____ x/day.

SPECIAL PROTOCOLS/NOTES: __Keep eyes looking forward._____

_____

_____

PATIENT NAME: _____DATE:_____

THERAPIST NAME:_____

Shoulder Flexion Push

PURPOSE: To strengthen shoulder muscles.

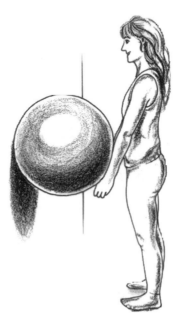

INSTRUCTION: Stand facing wall. Relax one arm down next to body (thumb facing wall). Place ball between wall and hand. Push hand into ball. Repeat with opposite side.

Hold: _____ second(s).   Repeat: _____ time(s).

Frequency: _____ x/day.

SPECIAL PROTOCOLS/NOTES: _____

_____

_____

PATIENT NAME: _____DATE:_____

THERAPIST NAME:_____

Shoulder Extension Push

PURPOSE: To strengthen shoulder muscles.

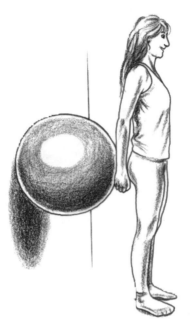

INSTRUCTION: Stand with back to wall. Relax one arm next to body (thumb facing forward). Place ball between wall and hand. Push hand into ball. Repeat with opposite side.

Hold: _____ second(s).   Repeat: _____ time(s).

Frequency: _____ x/day.

SPECIAL PROTOCOLS/NOTES: _____

_____

_____

PATIENT NAME: _____ DATE: _____

THERAPIST NAME: _____

Shoulder Internal Rotation Push

PURPOSE: To strengthen shoulder muscles.

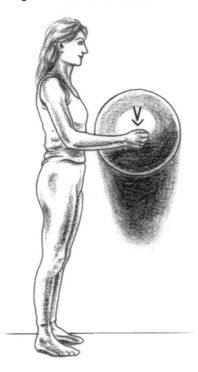

INSTRUCTION: Stand with side to wall. Place ball between wall and outside hand. Push hand into ball. Repeat with opposite side.

Hold: _____ second(s).   Repeat: _____ time(s).

Frequency: _____ x/day.

SPECIAL PROTOCOLS/NOTES: _____

_____

_____

PATIENT NAME: _____DATE:_____

THERAPIST NAME:_____

Shoulder External Rotation Push

PURPOSE: To strengthen shoulder muscles.

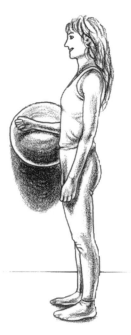

INSTRUCTION: Stand with side to wall. Place ball between inside hand and wall. Push ball into wall. Repeat with opposite side.

Hold: _____ second(s).   Repeat: _____ time(s).

Frequency: _____ x/day.

SPECIAL PROTOCOLS/NOTES: _____

_____

_____

PATIENT NAME: _____DATE:_____

THERAPIST NAME:_____

Shoulder Flexion with Ball against Wall

PURPOSE: To increase range of motion and strengthen shoulder muscles.

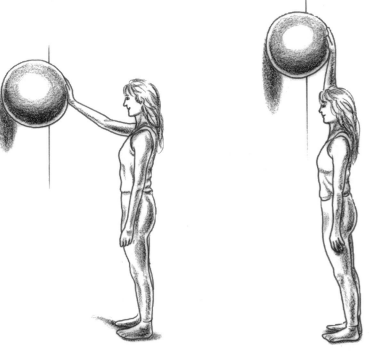

INSTRUCTION: Stand facing wall. Place ball between wall and hand. Roll ball up wall with hand. Step forward with both feet as ball rolls higher. Repeat with opposite side.

Hold: _____ second(s).   Repeat: _____ time(s).

Frequency: _____ x/day.

SPECIAL PROTOCOLS/NOTES: _____

_____

_____

PATIENT NAME: _____DATE:_____

THERAPIST NAME:_____

Shoulder Abduction with Ball against Wall

PURPOSE: To increase range of motion and strengthen shoulder muscles.

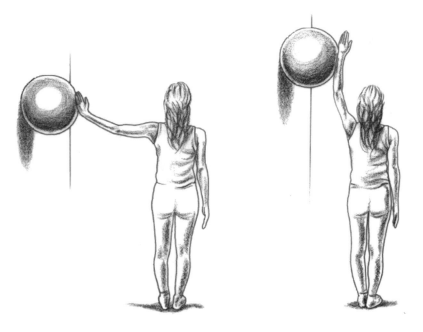

INSTRUCTION: Stand with side of body to wall. Place ball between wall and side of hand. Roll ball up with hand. Step toward wall with both feet as ball rolls up. Repeat with opposite side.

Hold: _____ second(s).   Repeat: _____ time(s).

Frequency: _____ x/day.

SPECIAL PROTOCOLS/NOTES: _____

_____

_____

PATIENT NAME: _____DATE:_____

THERAPIST NAME:_____

Knee Flexion/Extension

PURPOSE: To strengthen knee and leg muscles. To improve balance reactions.

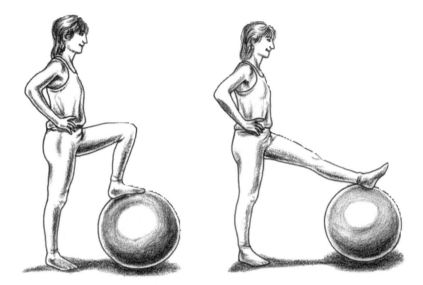

INSTRUCTION: Stand. Bend and lift knee. Place foot on ball. Extend leg out from body. Repeat with opposite side.

Hold: _____ second(s).   Repeat: _____ time(s).

Frequency: _____ x/day.

SPECIAL PROTOCOLS/NOTES: _____

_____

_____

PATIENT NAME: _____DATE:_____

THERAPIST NAME:_____

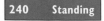

Write Alphabet with Foot

PURPOSE: To increase range of motion in ankles and knees. To improve balance reactions.

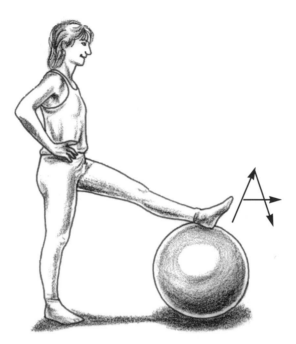

INSTRUCTION: Stand. Bend and lift one knee. Place foot on ball. Extend leg. Write alphabet with foot. Repeat with opposite side.

Hold: _____ second(s).   Repeat: _____ time(s).

Frequency: _____ x/day.

SPECIAL PROTOCOLS/NOTES: _____

_____

_____

PATIENT NAME: _____DATE:_____

THERAPIST NAME:_____

Hip Flexion/Extension

PURPOSE: To increase range of motion and strengthen hip muscles.

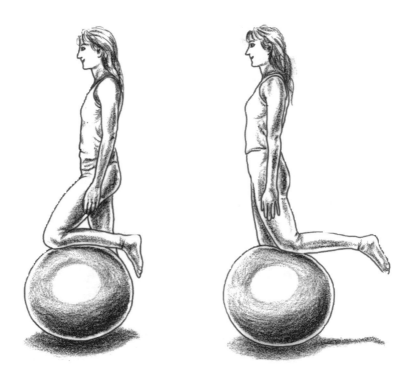

INSTRUCTION: Stand. Bend one knee and place on top of ball. Bend at hip and move ball forward. Extend hip and move ball backward. Repeat with opposite side.

Hold: _____ second(s).   Repeat: _____ time(s).

Frequency: _____ x/day.

SPECIAL PROTOCOLS/NOTES: _____

_____

_____

PATIENT NAME: _____ DATE:_____

THERAPIST NAME:_____

Hip Internal/External Rotation

PURPOSE: To increase range of motion and strengthen hip muscles.

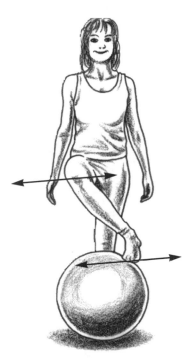

INSTRUCTION: Stand. Place foot on ball. Roll ball from side to side with foot. Allow knee to move in and out. Repeat with opposite side.

Hold: _____ second(s).   Repeat: _____ time(s).

Frequency: _____ x/day.

SPECIAL PROTOCOLS/NOTES: ___Knee should move in and out._____

_____

_____

PATIENT NAME: _____DATE:_____

THERAPIST NAME:_____

Partial Squats

PURPOSE: To strengthen buttock and leg muscles.

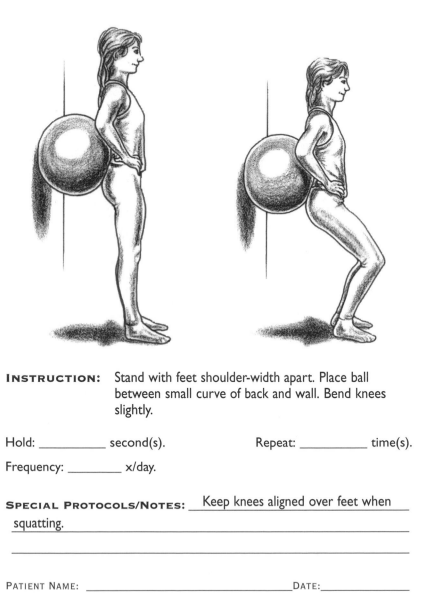

INSTRUCTION: Stand with feet shoulder-width apart. Place ball between small curve of back and wall. Bend knees slightly.

Hold: _____ second(s). Repeat: _____ time(s).

Frequency: _____ x/day.

SPECIAL PROTOCOLS/NOTES: ___Keep knees aligned over feet when___ squatting._____

_____

PATIENT NAME: _____DATE:_____

THERAPIST NAME:_____

Full Squats

PURPOSE: To strengthen buttock and leg muscles.

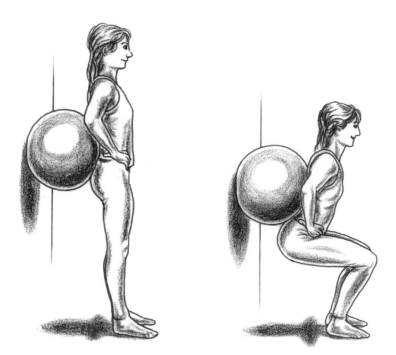

INSTRUCTION: Stand with feet shoulder-width apart. Place ball between small curve in back and wall. Bend knees.

Hold: _____ second(s).   Repeat: _____ time(s).

Frequency: _____ x/day.

SPECIAL PROTOCOLS/NOTES: ___Keep knees aligned over feet when___ squatting._____

_____

PATIENT NAME: _____DATE:_____

THERAPIST NAME:_____

Unilateral Squat

PURPOSE: To strengthen buttock and leg muscles.

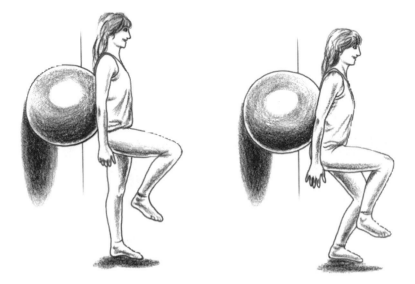

INSTRUCTION: Stand. Place ball between small curve of back and wall. Raise one knee toward ceiling. Bend opposite knee. Repeat with opposite side.

Hold: _____ second(s).   Repeat: _____ time(s).

Frequency: _____ x/day.

SPECIAL PROTOCOLS/NOTES: _____

_____

_____

PATIENT NAME: _____ DATE: _____

THERAPIST NAME: _____

Full Squat with Two Balls

PURPOSE: To strengthen knee and leg muscles. To stabilize mid back.

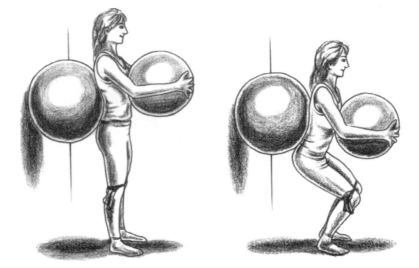

INSTRUCTION: Stand with ball against wall and small curve of back. Wrap resistive band around knees. Place second ball between arms. Bend knees.

Hold: _____ second(s).   Repeat: _____ time(s).

Frequency: _____ x/day.

SPECIAL PROTOCOLS/NOTES: _____Keep knees aligned over feet when____ squatting._____

_____

PATIENT NAME: _____DATE:_____

THERAPIST NAME:_____

Full Squat Facing Ball

PURPOSE: To strengthen buttock and leg muscles.

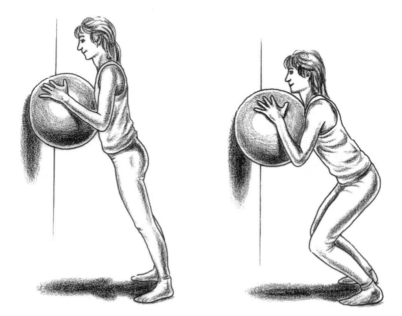

INSTRUCTION: Stand with feet shoulder-width apart. Place ball between chest and wall and lean into ball. Bend knees.

Hold: _____ second(s).   Repeat: _____ time(s).

Frequency: _____ x/day.

SPECIAL PROTOCOLS/NOTES: _Keep knees aligned over feet when_ squatting. _____

_____

PATIENT NAME: _____ DATE: _____

THERAPIST NAME: _____

Stoop Lift

PURPOSE: To strengthen arm, back, and leg muscles.

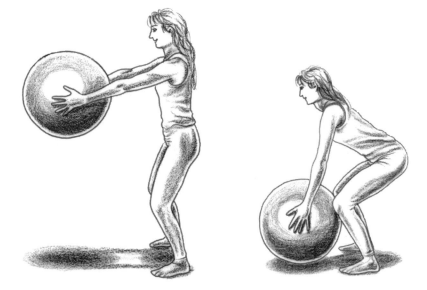

INSTRUCTION: Place ball between hands. Bend knees. Lower ball to floor and bend at waist. Keep eyes and chin level.

Hold: _____ second(s).   Repeat: _____ time(s).

Frequency: _____ x/day.

SPECIAL PROTOCOLS/NOTES: _____

_____

_____

PATIENT NAME: _____ DATE:_____

THERAPIST NAME:_____

Shoulder to Overhead Lift

PURPOSE: To strengthen arm, back, and leg muscles.

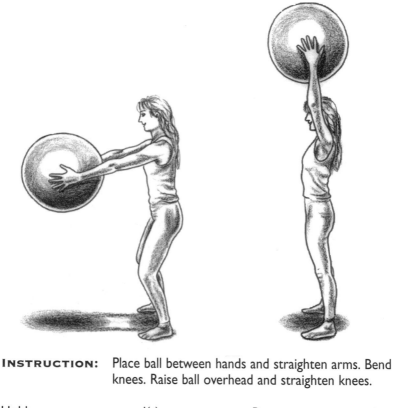

INSTRUCTION: Place ball between hands and straighten arms. Bend knees. Raise ball overhead and straighten knees.

Hold: _____ second(s).   Repeat: _____ time(s).

Frequency: _____ x/day.

SPECIAL PROTOCOLS/NOTES: _____

_____

_____

PATIENT NAME: _____ DATE:_____

THERAPIST NAME:_____

Stoop to Overhead Lift

PURPOSE: To strengthen arm, back, and leg muscles.

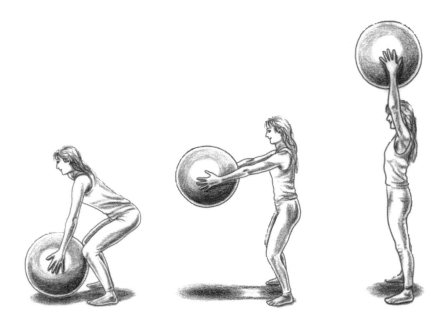

INSTRUCTION: Begin in stoop position with ball between hands. Shift weight backward and lift ball to shoulder height. Raise ball overhead.

Hold: _____ second(s).   Repeat: _____ time(s).

Frequency: _____ x/day.

SPECIAL PROTOCOLS/NOTES: _____

_____

_____

PATIENT NAME: _____ DATE: _____

THERAPIST NAME: _____

Lunge

PURPOSE: To strengthen arm and leg muscles.

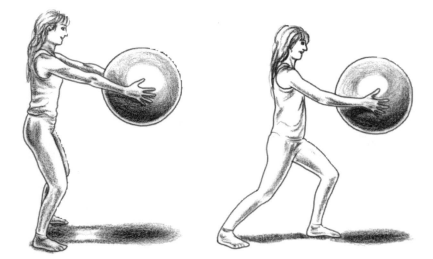

INSTRUCTION: Stand. Place ball between hands. Bend knees. Lunge forward with one leg. Repeat with opposite side.

Hold: _____ second(s). Repeat: _____ time(s).

Frequency: _____ x/day.

SPECIAL PROTOCOLS/NOTES: _____

_____

_____

PATIENT NAME: _____ DATE:_____

THERAPIST NAME:_____

The Glide

PURPOSE: To strengthen abdominal, arm, back, and leg muscles. To improve coordination and balance reactions.

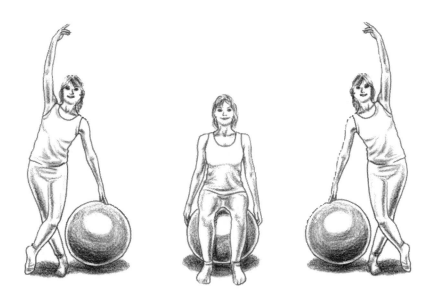

INSTRUCTION: Stand with right hand overhead and left hand touching ball at side. Cross left leg in front of right. In gliding motion, step sideways with left foot, bend knees, sit down on ball, and lower right arm. Cross right foot over left leg, raise left arm overhead, and stand up with right arm touching ball. Repeat in opposite direction.

Repeat: _____ time(s).   Frequency: _____ x/day.

SPECIAL PROTOCOLS/NOTES: _____

_____

_____

PATIENT NAME: _____DATE:_____

THERAPIST NAME:_____

Resistive Band Exercises

Wrist Flexion

PURPOSE: To strengthen wrist muscles.

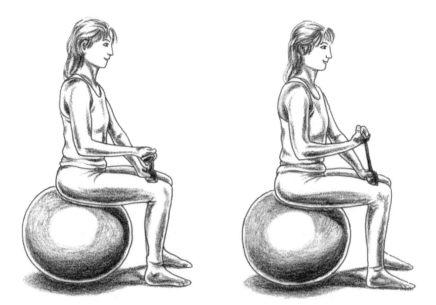

INSTRUCTION: Sit on ball in neutral position. Wrap resistive band around hands. Bend elbow with palm facing up. Bend wrist and raise up. Repeat with opposite side.

Hold: _____ second(s).   Repeat: _____ time(s).

Frequency: _____ x/day.

SPECIAL PROTOCOLS/NOTES: _____

_____

_____

PATIENT NAME: _____DATE:_____

THERAPIST NAME:_____

Wrist Extension

PURPOSE: To strengthen wrist muscles.

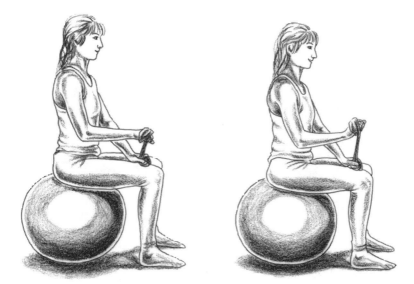

INSTRUCTION: Sit on ball in neutral position. Wrap resistive band around hands. Bend one elbow with palm facing down. Raise hand up. Repeat with opposite side.

Hold: _____ second(s).   Repeat: _____ time(s).

Frequency: _____ x/day.

SPECIAL PROTOCOLS/NOTES: _____

_____

_____

PATIENT NAME: _____DATE:_____

THERAPIST NAME:_____

Elbow Flexion

PURPOSE: To strengthen arm muscles.

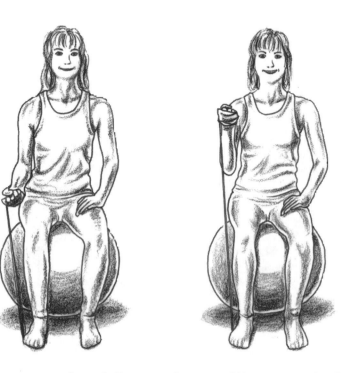

INSTRUCTION: Sit on ball in neutral position. Wrap resistive band around hand. Place end of resistive band under foot. Bend one elbow with palm up. Repeat with opposite side.

Hold: _____ second(s).   Repeat: _____ time(s).

Frequency: _____ x/day.

SPECIAL PROTOCOLS/NOTES: _____

_____

_____

PATIENT NAME: _____DATE:_____

THERAPIST NAME:_____

Elbow Extension

PURPOSE: To strengthen back of arm muscles.

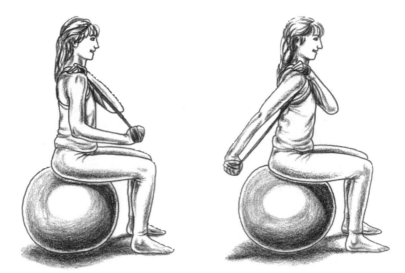

INSTRUCTION: Sit on ball in neutral position. Wrap resistive band around hands. Bend one elbow. Extend other arm behind back. Repeat with opposite side.

Hold: _____ second(s).   Repeat: _____ time(s).

Frequency: _____ x/day.

SPECIAL PROTOCOLS/NOTES: _____

_____

_____

PATIENT NAME: _____DATE:_____

THERAPIST NAME:_____

Shoulder Internal Rotation

PURPOSE: To strengthen shoulder muscles.

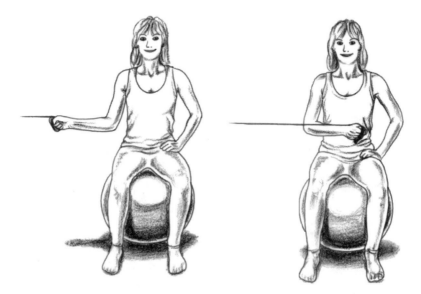

INSTRUCTION: Tie knot in resistive band and shut in doorway. Sit on ball in neutral position. Wrap band around hand. Bend elbow and bring hand in toward abdomen. Repeat with opposite hand.

Hold: _____ second(s).   Repeat: _____ time(s).

Frequency: _____ x/day.

SPECIAL PROTOCOLS/NOTES: _____

_____

_____

PATIENT NAME: _____ DATE: _____

THERAPIST NAME: _____

Shoulder
External Rotation

PURPOSE: To strengthen shoulder muscles.

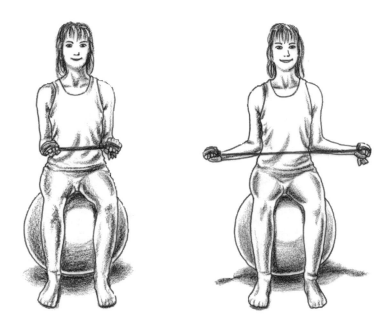

INSTRUCTION: Sit on ball in neutral position. Wrap resistive band
around hands. Bend elbows. Move hands out away
from body. Keep elbows next to body.

Hold: _____ second(s).   Repeat: _____ time(s).

Frequency: _____ x/day.

SPECIAL PROTOCOLS/NOTES: _____

_____

_____

PATIENT NAME: _____DATE:_____

THERAPIST NAME:_____

Shoulder
Protraction/Retraction

PURPOSE: To strengthen shoulder muscles.

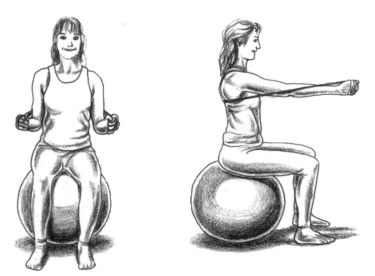

INSTRUCTION: Sit on ball in neutral position. Wrap resistive band around hands. Loop band behind back. Bend elbows and push hands forward.

Hold: _____ second(s).   Repeat: _____ time(s).

Frequency: _____ x/day.

SPECIAL PROTOCOLS/NOTES: _____

_____

_____

PATIENT NAME: _____DATE:_____

THERAPIST NAME:_____

Shoulder Protraction across Body

PURPOSE: To strengthen shoulder muscles.

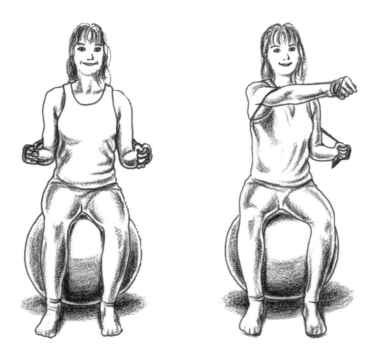

INSTRUCTION: Sit on ball in neutral position. Wrap resistive band around hands. Loop band around back. Bend elbows. Push one hand forward and across body. Repeat with opposite side.

Hold: _____ second(s).   Repeat: _____ time(s).

Frequency: _____ x/day.

SPECIAL PROTOCOLS/NOTES: _____

_____

_____

PATIENT NAME: _____ DATE:_____

THERAPIST NAME:_____

Shoulder Horizontal Abduction

PURPOSE: To strengthen arm muscles.

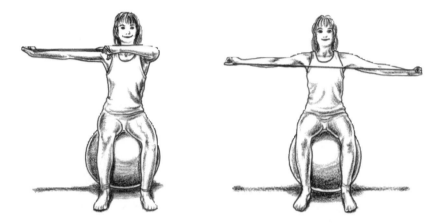

INSTRUCTION: Sit on ball in neutral position. Wrap resistive band around hands. Begin with left hand on right shoulder. Pull left arm across body. Repeat with opposite side.

Hold: _____ second(s).   Repeat: _____ time(s).

Frequency: _____ x/day.

SPECIAL PROTOCOLS/NOTES: _____

_____

_____

PATIENT NAME: _____ DATE: _____

THERAPIST NAME: _____

Shoulder Abduction

PURPOSE: To strengthen shoulder muscles.

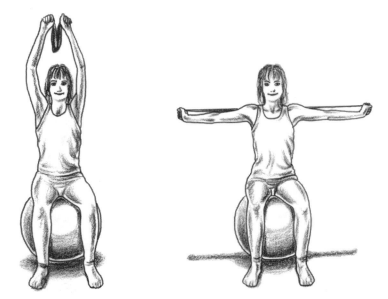

INSTRUCTION: Sit on ball in neutral position. Wrap resistive band around hands. Raise arms overhead. Lower arms to shoulder height and pull band behind head.

Hold: _____ second(s).   Repeat: _____ time(s).

Frequency: _____ x/day.

SPECIAL PROTOCOLS/NOTES: _____

_____

_____

PATIENT NAME: _____DATE:_____

THERAPIST NAME:_____

Shoulder PNF Diagonal

PURPOSE: To strengthen shoulder muscles.

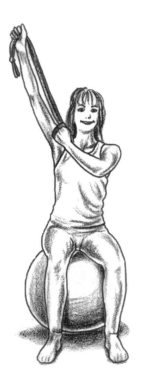 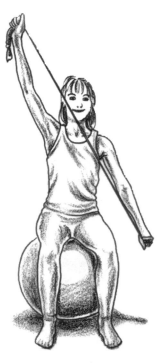

INSTRUCTION: Sit on ball. Wrap resistive band around hands. Raise right arm overhead. Place left hand on right shoulder. Extend left arm down toward left hip. Repeat with opposite side.

Hold: _____ second(s). Repeat: _____ time(s).

Frequency: _____ x/day.

SPECIAL PROTOCOLS/NOTES: _____

_____

_____

PATIENT NAME: _____DATE:_____

THERAPIST NAME:_____

Plantar Flexion

PURPOSE: To strengthen calf muscles.

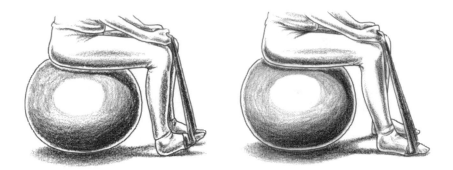

INSTRUCTION: Sit on ball in neutral position. Wrap resistive band around foot. Pull toes up and push down. Repeat with opposite foot.

Hold: _____ second(s).   Repeat: _____ time(s).

Frequency: _____ x/day.

SPECIAL PROTOCOLS/NOTES: _____

_____

_____

PATIENT NAME: _____ DATE:_____

THERAPIST NAME:_____

Dorsiflexion

PURPOSE: To strengthen ankle muscles.

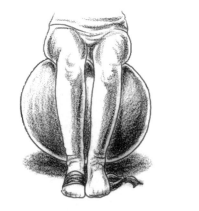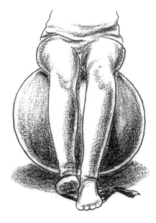

INSTRUCTION: Sit on ball in neutral position. Loop resistive band around right foot. Step on band with left foot. Raise right foot up toward ceiling. Repeat with opposite foot.

Hold: _____ second(s).   Repeat: _____ time(s).

Frequency: _____ x/day.

SPECIAL PROTOCOLS/NOTES: _____

_____

_____

PATIENT NAME: _____ DATE:_____

THERAPIST NAME:_____

Hip Adduction/Abduction

PURPOSE: To strengthen inner and outer thigh muscles.

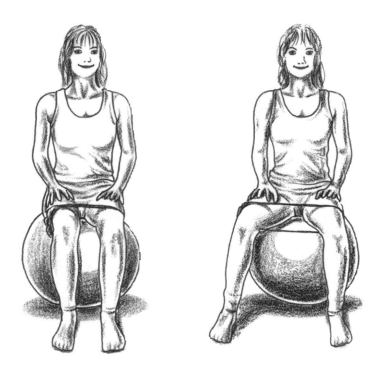

INSTRUCTION: Sit on ball in neutral position. Wrap resistive band around knees. Move knee and foot out. Repeat with opposite side.

Hold: _____ second(s).   Repeat: _____ time(s).

Frequency: _____ x/day.

SPECIAL PROTOCOLS/NOTES: _____

_____

_____

PATIENT NAME: _____ DATE: _____

THERAPIST NAME: _____

Hip Flexion

PURPOSE: To strengthen hip muscles.

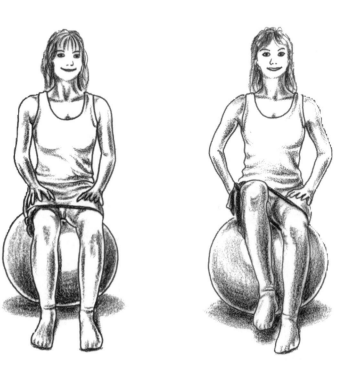

INSTRUCTION: Sit on ball in neutral position. Wrap resistive band around knees. Raise one knee toward ceiling. Repeat with opposite knee.

Hold: _____ second(s).   Repeat: _____ time(s).

Frequency: _____ x/day.

SPECIAL PROTOCOLS/NOTES: _____

_____

_____

PATIENT NAME: _____ DATE: _____

THERAPIST NAME: _____

Prone Shoulder Flexion

PURPOSE: To strengthen arm and neck muscles.

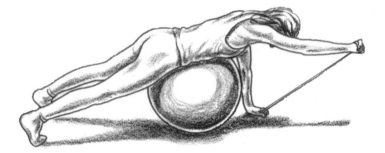

INSTRUCTION: Lie with abdomen on ball. Wrap resistive band around hands. Place both hands in front of ball. Raise one arm overhead. Repeat with opposite arm.

Hold: _____ second(s).   Repeat: _____ time(s).

Frequency: _____ x/day.

SPECIAL PROTOCOLS/NOTES: Do not lift arm so high back rotates.

_____

_____

PATIENT NAME: _____DATE:_____

THERAPIST NAME:_____

Prone Shoulder
Flexion/Extension

PURPOSE: To strengthen arm, back, and neck muscles.

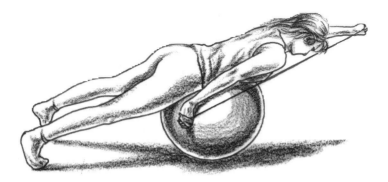

INSTRUCTION: Lie with abdomen on ball. Wrap resistive band around
hands. Extend one arm overhead with the other arm
extended back. Repeat with opposite side.

Hold: _____ second(s).   Repeat: _____ time(s).

Frequency: _____ x/day.

SPECIAL PROTOCOLS/NOTES: _____

_____

_____

PATIENT NAME: _____DATE:_____

THERAPIST NAME:_____

Prone Shoulder Abduction

PURPOSE: To strengthen arm, back, neck, and shoulder muscles.

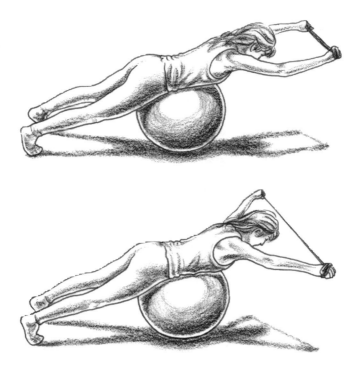

INSTRUCTION: Lie with abdomen on ball. Wrap resistive band around hands. Raise arms overhead. Move arms out and away from body.

Hold: _____ second(s).   Repeat: _____ time(s).

Frequency: _____ x/day.

SPECIAL PROTOCOLS/NOTES: _____

_____

_____

PATIENT NAME: _____DATE:_____

THERAPIST NAME:_____

Unilateral Shoulder Flexion
in Bridge Position

PURPOSE: To strengthen arm, back, leg, and abdominal muscles. To improve balance reactions.

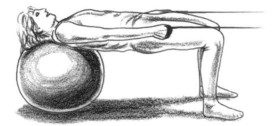

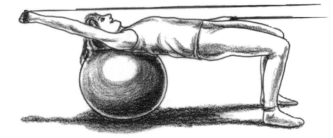

INSTRUCTION: Tie a knot in resistive band and shut in door. Lie on ball in bridge position. Place one piece of band in each hand. Alternate raising hands overhead.

Hold: _____ second(s).   Repeat: _____ time(s).

Frequency: _____ x/day.

SPECIAL PROTOCOLS/NOTES: _____

_____

_____

PATIENT NAME: _____ DATE:_____

THERAPIST NAME:_____

1-800-530-6878. © Copyright Executive Physical Therapy, 1994.
Reproduction of this page is permissible for instructional use only.

Unilateral Shoulder Extension in Bridge Position

PURPOSE: To strengthen arm, back, leg, and abdominal muscles. To improve balance reactions.

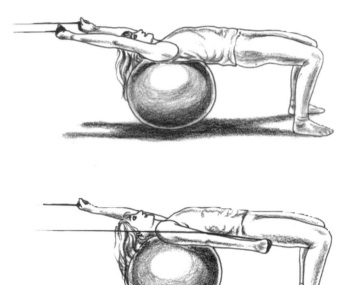

INSTRUCTION: Tie a knot in resistive band and shut in door. Lie on ball in bridge position. Raise hands overhead. Place piece of band in each hand. Alternate lowering one hand to side of body.

Hold: _____ second(s).   Repeat: _____ time(s).

Frequency: _____ x/day.

SPECIAL PROTOCOLS/NOTES: _____

_____

_____

PATIENT NAME: _____ **DATE:**_____

THERAPIST NAME:_____

Hand Exercises

Tip Pinch

PURPOSE: To increase pinch strength between thumb and index finger.

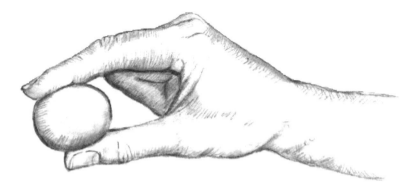

INSTRUCTION: Place ball between thumb and index finger. Squeeze ball. Repeat with opposite hand.

Hold: _____ second(s).   Repeat: _____ time(s).

Frequency: _____ x/day.

SPECIAL PROTOCOLS/NOTES: _____

_____

_____

PATIENT NAME: _____DATE:_____

THERAPIST NAME:_____

Three Jaw Grasp

PURPOSE: To increase pinch strength between thumb, index, and middle finger.

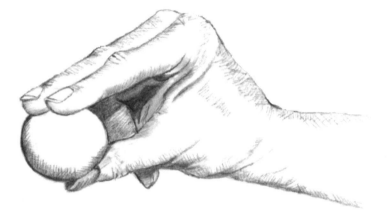

INSTRUCTION: Place ball between thumb, index, and middle finger. Squeeze ball. Repeat with opposite hand.

Hold: _____ second(s).   Repeat: _____ time(s).

Frequency: _____ x/day.

SPECIAL PROTOCOLS/NOTES: ___May bend knuckles if indicated.___

_____

_____

PATIENT NAME: _____DATE:_____

THERAPIST NAME:_____

Lateral Pinch

PURPOSE: To increase pinch strength between thumb and index finger.

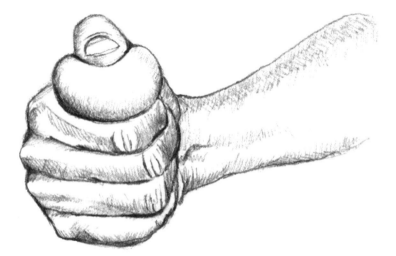

INSTRUCTION: Place ball between thumb and index finger. Squeeze ball. Repeat with opposite hand.

Hold: _____ second(s).   Repeat: _____ time(s).

Frequency: _____ x/day.

SPECIAL PROTOCOLS/NOTES: _____

_____

_____

PATIENT NAME: _____DATE:_____

THERAPIST NAME:_____

Ball Squeeze with Hand

PURPOSE: To strengthen flexor muscles in hand.

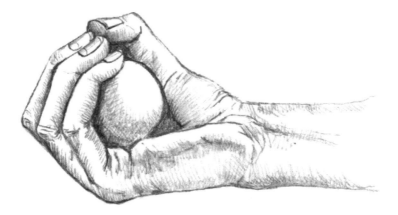

INSTRUCTION: Place ball in hand. Squeeze ball with fingers and thumb. Repeat with opposite hand.

Hold: _____ second(s).   Repeat: _____ time(s).

Frequency: _____ x/day.

SPECIAL PROTOCOLS/NOTES: _____

_____

_____

PATIENT NAME: _____DATE:_____

THERAPIST NAME:_____

Thumb
Extension/Flexion/Opposition

PURPOSE: To increase range of motion and strength in thumb.

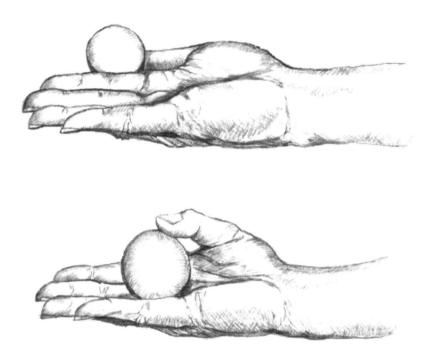

INSTRUCTION: Place ball on inside of thumb. Roll ball toward pinky
finger. Return to starting position. Repeat with
opposite hand.

Hold: _____ second(s).   Repeat: _____ time(s).

Frequency: _____ x/day.

SPECIAL PROTOCOLS/NOTES: _____

_____

_____

PATIENT NAME: _____ DATE:_____

THERAPIST NAME:_____

Finger Adduction

PURPOSE: To increase strength in inside of fingers.

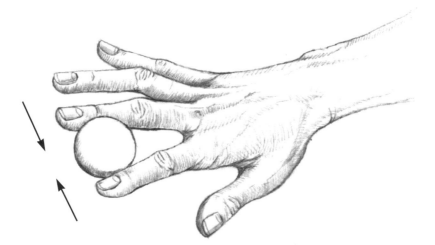

INSTRUCTION: Place ball between index and middle finger. Squeeze
ball. Repeat exercise between middle finger and ring
finger, and ring finger and pinky finger. Repeat with
opposite hand.

Hold: _____ second(s).   Repeat: _____ time(s).

Frequency: _____ x/day.

SPECIAL PROTOCOLS/NOTES: _____

_____

_____

PATIENT NAME: _____ DATE: _____

THERAPIST NAME: _____

Finger Scissor

PURPOSE: To increase range of motion, strength, and coordination in fingers.

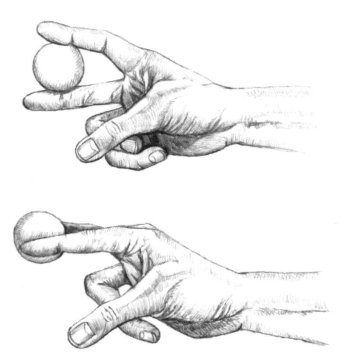

INSTRUCTION: Place ball between index finger and middle finger. Rotate ball clockwise and counter-clockwise. Repeat exercise between middle finger and ring finger, and ring finger and pinky finger. Repeat with opposite hand.

Repeat: _____ time(s).   Frequency: _____ x/day.

SPECIAL PROTOCOLS/NOTES: _____

_____

_____

PATIENT NAME: _____ DATE:_____

THERAPIST NAME:_____

Metacarpal Phalangeal Extension

PURPOSE: To increase strength at base of fingers.

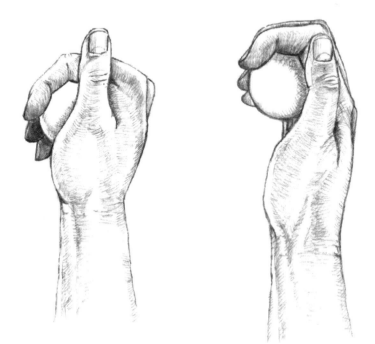

INSTRUCTION: Place ball between flexed fingers. Extend joint at base of fingers. Return to starting position. Repeat with opposite hand.

Hold: _____ second(s).   Repeat: _____ time(s).

Frequency: _____ x/day.

SPECIAL PROTOCOLS/NOTES: _____

_____

_____

PATIENT NAME: _____ DATE:_____

THERAPIST NAME:_____

Radial Thumb Flick

PURPOSE: To increase range of motion, strength, and coordination in thumb.

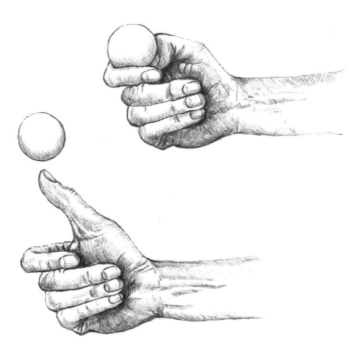

INSTRUCTION: Place ball on top of thumb. Flick ball upward with thumb. Repeat with opposite hand.

Repeat: _____ time(s).   Frequency: _____ x/day.

SPECIAL PROTOCOLS/NOTES: __Keep wrist in neutral position._____

_____

_____

PATIENT NAME: _____ DATE:_____

THERAPIST NAME:_____

Radial Abduction with Palm Facing Down

PURPOSE: To increase range of motion, strength, and coordination in thumb.

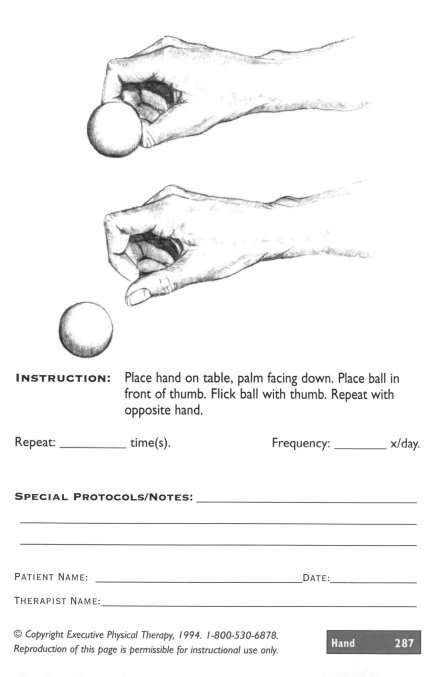

INSTRUCTION: Place hand on table, palm facing down. Place ball in front of thumb. Flick ball with thumb. Repeat with opposite hand.

Repeat: _____ time(s).   Frequency: _____ x/day.

SPECIAL PROTOCOLS/NOTES: _____

_____

_____

PATIENT NAME: _____DATE:_____

THERAPIST NAME:_____

Rotate Two Balls in Hand

PURPOSE: To strengthen thumb and finger muscles. To improve coordination.

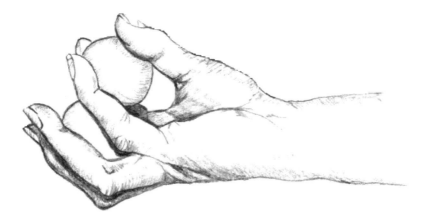

INSTRUCTION: Place two balls in hand. Rotate the two balls between thumb and fingers. Repeat with opposite hand.

Repeat: _____ time(s).   Frequency: _____ x/day.

SPECIAL PROTOCOLS/NOTES: _____

_____

_____

PATIENT NAME: _____DATE:_____

THERAPIST NAME:_____

INDEX

Suggested Reading

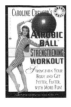

Creager, Caroline Corning. *The Airobic Ball*™ *Strengthening Workout*. Berthoud, Colo .: Executive Physical Therapy, Inc. 1994

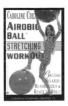

Creager, Caroline Corning. *The Airobic Ball*™ *Stretching Workout*. Berthoud, Colo.: Executive Physical Therapy, Inc. 1995

Creager, Caroline Corning. *Therapeutic Exercises Using the Foam Rollers*. Berthoud, Colo.: Executive Physical Therapy, Inc. 1996

∽∾

Hosting a Swiss Ball Course
by Caroline Corning Creager, PT

If you are interested in hosting a Swiss Ball course, please call 1-800-530-OTPT or write to Executive Physical Therapy, Inc. at the address listed below.

∽∾

Questions/New Ideas or Exercises

If you have any questions or a Swiss Ball exercise that you love and would like to have included in a future edition, please write:

Executive Physical Therapy, Inc.
P.O. Box 1319, Berthoud, CO 80513